D1764888

Nursing Practice in Multiple Sclerosis: A Core Curriculum

Kathleen Costello, RN, MS, CRNP, MSCN
Maryland Center for Multiple Sclerosis
University of Maryland
Baltimore, Maryland

June Halper, MSCN, ANP, FAAN
Gimbel Multiple Sclerosis Center,
Consortium of Multiple Sclerosis Centers (CMSC)
Teaneck, New Jersey

and

Colleen Harris, RN, MN, MSCN
Multiple Sclerosis Clinic
Foothills Hospital
Calgary, Alberta

Demos

Demos Medical Publishing, 386 Park Avenue South, New York, New York 10016

Library of Congress Cataloging-in-Publication Data

Costello, Kathleen.
  Nursing practice in multiple sclerosis : a core curriculum / Kathleen Costello, June Halper, and Colleen Harris.
    p. ; cm.
  ISBN 1-888799-76-5 (pbk.)
  1. Multiple sclerosis—Nursing.
  [DNLM: 1. Multiple Sclerosis—nursing. WL 360 C84 ln 2003]   I. Halper, June.
II. Harris ,Colleen.   III. Title.
  RC377 .C66 2003
  610.73'69—dc21

                                    200711505   2002151624
                                    2-6-03

Printed in Canada

Visit the Demos Medical Publishing web site at www.demosmedpub.com

Dedication

This work is dedicated to all of our MS patients and families who have taught us the meaning of strength and hope in the face of adversity, and to our MS team throughout the world.

In memory of Morris Halper, M.D., whose spirit lives on in the work of June Halper.

Acknowledgments

We would like to acknowledge Dr. Diana M. Schneider for her support of MS nursing and her skill and editorial support in the development of this resource for MS nurses.

    We would also like to thank TevaNeuroscience, especially Judith K. Katterhenrich, for their encouragement and collaborative spirit.

Contents

Preface: Kathleen Costello, RN, MS, CRNP, MSCN   v

**Background Information for Nursing Practice
in Multiple Sclerosis**

1. The History of Multiple Sclerosis Care   1

2. Domains of Multiple Sclerosis Nursing Practice   7

3. Change Theory and Its Application in
   Multiple Sclerosis Nursing   11

4. Multiple Sclerosis Nurses' Code of Ethics   13

The Diagnosis of Multiple Sclerosis

5. Epidemiology   17

6. The Complete Neurologic Examination   21

7. Magnetic Resonance Imaging (MRI)   127

8. Determining the Diagnosis and Prognosis
   of Multiple Sclerosis   31

Management of the Disease Process

9. The Immune System and Its Role in Multiple Sclerosis   39

10. Disease-Altering Therapies   43

Functional Alterations: Physical Domains

11. The Symptom Chain in Multiple Sclerosis   51

12. The Multiple Sclerosis Care Team   65

13. Bladder Dysfunction   69

14. Bowel Elimination and Continence   75

15. The Nurse's Role in Advanced Multiple Sclerosis   81

Functional Alterations: Personal Domain

16. Psychosocial Implications   85

17. Financial and Vocational Concerns   87

Shaping Multiple Sclerosis Nursing Practice

18. Primary Care Needs   91

19. The Nurse's Role in Multiple Sclerosis Research   95

20. Study Guide in Multiple Sclerosis   99

21. Case Studies   101

22. Certification Study Questions   113

Preface

Multiple sclerosis is a lifelong, potentially disabling disease of the central nervous system that affects the white matter tracts of the central nervous system in a sporadic and unpredictable manner. The disease produces inflammation and demyelination of the white matter, as well as varying amounts of damage and destruction to the underlying axon. The onset of disease is most often in early adulthood. Individuals experience a myriad of symptoms with likely progression of disability over time. Symptoms may include fatigue, visual disturbances, sensory changes, incoordination, pain, tremor, elimination dysfunction, and cognitive impairment. Symptoms usually occur as relapses early in the disease, or as symptoms that appear over 24–48 hours and recede to some extent over weeks to months. After a decade or so, many individuals experience fewer relapses, but in their place is a slow progression of MS symptoms that often leads to increased functional disability over time. A small percentage of patients will experience progression from the onset of the disease and experience progressive mobility impairment over time.

MS invades every aspect of life, and patients as well as families can be severely affected. Patients and families experience a sense of loss, both real and perceived. The disease can adversely impact the roles of provider, spouse, parent, friend, and employee. There are emotional consequences of the disease as well as physical ones. As the disease is one for life, individuals and families will have multiple needs throughout their lives. They will need emotional support, education, symptom management, adaptation to changes, adaptive equipment, supportive care, and perhaps even end of life care.

Nursing is a critical element in meeting the multiple needs of the MS patient and family. MS nurses have evolved from home-based care providers giving support to the disabled person to certified MS nurses and advanced practice nurses who must be well educated in the disease process and the available treatments. In addition, MS nurses must be sensitive to and supportive of the emotional needs of those affected by the disease. MS nurses must provide appropriate education regarding the disease process, treatment regimes, symptom management, and community resources.

As MS knows few borders, MS nurses are needed throughout the world. Nurses need to share experiences and knowledge to support MS patients and families as well as each other. Through the vision of June Halper, MSCN, ANP, FAAN, the International Organization of Multiple Sclerosis Nurses (IOMSN) was founded in 1997. Its mission is to establish and perpetuate a specialized branch of nursing in multiple sclerosis; to establish standards of nursing care in multiple sclerosis; to support multiple sclerosis nursing research; to educate the healthcare community about the disease; and to disseminate this knowledge throughout the world. The ultimate goal of the IOMSN is to improve the lives of everyone affected by multiple sclerosis through the provision of appropriate healthcare services.

This IOMSN determined that the expertise of the MS nurse needed to be developed and recognized. To that end an international certification board, separate from the IOMSN, was established and a certification process was developed. The first MS nursing certification exam was given on June 5, 2002 in Chicago, Illinois. Over 100 nurses from around the world sat for this exam. Prior to the exam several review courses were held in various locations. It was clear following the review courses that a tremendous amount of knowledge is needed to be an "expert" in MS nursing.

This core curriculum summarizes in outline form the basic concepts of multiple sclerosis and MS nursing. Each chapter provides relevant information as well as references for further study. Readers will learn about the history of MS, as well as the current theories regarding the immunologic basis for the disease. Pharmacologic strategies that include treatment for acute attacks, immunomodulating therapies, and symptomatic therapies are discussed, as are nonpharmacologic interventions.

This text provides the reader with essential information about multiple sclerosis and its management. It is an excellent review for those interested in MS nursing certification, and an excellent resource and reference for the MS nurse. Through the dedicated efforts of June Halper, this core curriculum is available to all of us involved with the care of persons with MS.

Kathleen Costello, RN, MS, CRNP, MSCN
President, International Organization of
Multiple Sclerosis Nurses (IOMSN)

Chapter 1

The History of Multiple Sclerosis Care

Objectives:
Upon completion of this chapter, the learner will:

◆ Identify the evolution of knowledge that has impacted the care of people with multiple sclerosis (MS)
◆ Discuss turning points in the definition of MS
◆ Describe the networks in MS care

■ Multiple sclerosis (MS) is a common neurologic disease of young adults. It affects people in the prime of their lives with unpredictability and uncertainty.

■ In recent decades the hallmark of disease progression has been altered due to disease-modifying therapies for relapsing forms of the disease.

■ It has been known as a peculiar disease state (Robert Carswell), a gray degeneration of the cord (Jean Cruveilhier), and insular sclerosis (William Moxon and William Osler).

■ Disseminated sclerosis was a term used in the early part of the twentieth century.

■ The name "multiple sclerosis" is a derivation from the German "multiple sklerose."

■ Early cases were:
  A. Saint Lidwina van Schiedam
  B. Halla, the drummer Bock, and William Brown, a Hudson Bay official
  C. Sir Augustus d'Este
  D. Heinrich Heine
  E. Margaret Gatty

F. W.N.P. Barbellion
- An early monograph on MS was written by Charles Prosper Ollivier.
- Other writings on MS were by Robert Carswell, Jean Cruveilhier, Marshall Hall, and others. These included anatomic depictions of autopsy findings and the description included a clinical history.
- Jean-Martin Charcot framed the disease and thoroughly described the clinical and pathologic features of MS in 1868. He added to the observations of Carswell, Cruveilhier, and the German physician von Frerichs with his own, calling the disease *le sclerose en plaques* or scarring in patches.
- In 1873, Dr. Moxon in England characterized the disease based on observations.
- In 1878, Dr. Ranvier discovered myelin.
- For over 100 years, physicians were frustrated trying to identify the cause of MS. Theories of causation ranged from infection to genetics, vascular problems, and immunologic deficits.
- In 1916, Dr. Dawson at the University of Edinburgh in Scotland used a microscope to describe inflammation around the blood vessels and the damage to the myelin with a clarity and thoroughness that has never been improved. Little was known about the brain's function, so the meaning of these changes was only a guess.
- In 1919, abnormalities in cerebrospinal fluid (CSF) were observed. The significance was unknown.
- In 1925, the first electrical recording of nerve transmission was made by Lord Edgar Douglas Adrian. The science of electrophysiology established techniques needed to study nerves.
- In 1928, myelin was studied under a microscope; oligodendrocytes (cells that produce myelin) were discovered.
- In 1935, Dr. Rivers at the Rockefeller Institute in New York reproduced the autoimmune response classically seen in MS. An animal model for MS was developed called *experimental allergic encephalomyelitis* (EAE).
- Dietary modification was studied with no conclusive evidence of benefit.
- Alternative or complementary therapies emerged as a frequently used supplement or a substitute for conventional treatments.
- In 1946, Sylvia Lawry founded the National Multiple Sclerosis Society in New York City, which has expanded into a worldwide

MS Network of MS Societies. Services and programs include a wide range of patient and family services, basic and psychosocial research, and MS education. NMSS and the Canadian MS Society cover North America with a wide range of programs and services.

- Dr. Kabat at Columbia University received the first NMSS grant to study MS.
- Dr. Salk received an NMSS grant to study the immunology of MS.
- In 1950, NMSS helped to establish a new division of the National Institute of Health (NIH), the National Institute for Neurologic Disorders and Stroke (NINDS).
- In 1967, Ms. Lawry founded the International Federation of MS Societies, now the Multiple Sclerosis International Federation (MSIF).
- In 1969, the first successful clinical trial in the treatment of MS was held.
  A. Placebo controlled
  B. New rating scales and diagnostic standards used
  C. Patients were given ACTH
- In the 1970s, research produced useful results.
  A. Scientists studying EAE suspected myelin protein fragments prevented the disease
  B. A mixture of the fragments was used to treat animals and then humans with MS (copolymer 1)
  C. Steroids were now widely used to suppress immune response
  D. In 1978, computed tomography (CAT) scanning was first used for patients with MS
  E. First experiments with interferons demonstrated their immune-modulating effects
- The 1980s saw the beginnings of major clinical trials in MS using immunomodulators, such as interferons and glatiramer acetate (copolymer 1).
- Dr. Young performed the first magnetic resonance imaging (MRI) on a patient with MS.
- In 1984, it became apparent that MRI can visualize MS attacks in the brain, including many that did not manifest symptoms.
- In 1993, FDA approved Betaseron® (IFN-beta 1b) for relapsing remitting MS (R-R MS).

- In 1996, Avonex® (IFN-beta 1a) was approved for R-R MS.
- In 1996, Copaxone® (glatiramer acetate) was approved for R-R MS.
- In 1986, the Consortium of Multiple Sclerosis Centers (CMSC) was founded. The CMSC is the largest organization of MS health professionals in the world. It holds annual and regional meetings, consensus conferences, and training programs for MS professionals. It has a journal (*International Journal of MS Care*) and a newsletter (*The MS Exchange*). The CMSC Foundation funds scholarships and fellowships in MS training; the CMSC NARCOMS project has a large patient database to increase understanding of MS and its ramifications. Many studies have used the database.
- In 1991 Rehabilitation in Multiple Sclerosis (RIMS), a European network, was founded. The European Committee on Treatment and Research in MS (ECTRIMS) was founded shortly thereafter. ACTRIMS, the North American counterpart, was established followed by LACTRIMS, a Latin American organization representing Central and South America.
- In 1997, the International Organization of MS Nurses (IOMSN) was founded. The Goals and Strategies of the IOMSN are to:
A. Facilitate the development of a specialized branch of nursing in MS:
  1. Develop and maintain a mechanism by which members can share information on practice positions and resources
  2. Establish the IOMSN as a forum for discussion and collaboration on issues that concern MS nurses
  3. Serve as a resource for external organizations related to MS practice issues
  4. Promote the acknowledgment of the contribution of IOMSN as the pre-eminent organization of MS nurses
  5. Participate with other nursing organizations involved in MS care or related fields
  6. Share information on research activities among members
B. Establish standards of nursing care in MS:
  1. Develop minimal standards of nursing practice in MS
  2. Facilitate the development of a core curriculum for MS nursing to disseminate this information
  3. Identify specific domains of MS nursing and define basic roles and responsibilities in each domain

C. Support multiple sclerosis nursing research, basic research, and clinical trials:
  1. Encourage research activities that contribute to the development of a sound theoretical basis for MS practice
  2. Recommend research topics for educational sessions at IOMSN meetings for dissemination of evidence-based information
  3. Develop and implement nursing research
  4. Disseminate MS nursing research findings through publications and educational activities
D. Educate the healthcare community about MS:
  1. Promote communication among the IOMSN membership via the newsletter, web site, and other venues
  2. Facilitate internal and external communication about MS care and research

- Multiple Sclerosis International Credentialing Board (MSNICB) was founded in 2001
  A. The MSNICB is responsible for the development and administration of the Certification examination in MS nursing.
  B. The International Organization of Multiple Sclerosis Nurses (IOMSN) endorses the concept of voluntary certification by examination for all nursing professionals providing care in MS. Those who work or have worked in this specialty and meet eligibility requirements may be candidates to take this examination. Certification focuses specifically on the individual and is an indication of knowledge and skills and MS practice. MS nursing certification provides formal recognition of a level of knowledge in the field and promotes the delivery of safe and effective practice in the domains of Clinical Practice (disease course and classifications, epidemiology and distribution); Advocacy (ethical practice, negotiating the healthcare system, empowerment, knowledge of community resources, patient rights, consultation expertise); Education (principles of teaching/learning, health promotion and change theory, special populations, professional development); and Research (evidence-based practice, protection of human subjects, research terminology and process).

C. All candidates must be licensed nursing professionals with at least two years' experience in MS. Candidates must also agree to adhere to the IOMSN Code of Ethics.

D. The basic content of the examination covers:
  1. Basic concepts of MS (disease course classification, pathophysiology of MS, diagnostic process)
  2. Pharmacologic and nonpharmacologic treatment
  3. Symptom management
  4. Psychosocial intervention
  5. Research and education initiatives
  6. Patient advocacy

ADDITIONAL READING

Murray TJ. "The History of Multiple Sclerosis." In: Burks JS, Johnson KP, eds., *Multiple Sclerosis: Diagnosis, Medical Management, and Rehabilitation.* New York: Demos Medical Publishing, 2000; 1-35.

Polman CH, et al. *Multiple Sclerosis: The Guide to Treatment and Management*, 5th edition. New York: Demos Medical Publishing, 2001.

Halper J. The Founding of IOMSN and MSNICB. Personal Communication, 2002.

Chapter 2

Domains of Multiple Sclerosis Nursing Practice

> **Objectives:**
> Upon completion of this chapter, the learner will:
>
> ◆ List the four domains of MS nursing
> ◆ Describe nursing activities related to the core of care
> ◆ Cite professional responsibilities required to sustain the MS nursing role

- Nursing domains are considered the full range of nursing practice that may be called into use to serve the MS patient and the family.
- MS practice domains are broad areas of accountability.
- Broad areas of practice include the full range of knowledge, skills, and tasks of MS nursing responsibility.
- The domains of MS nursing include:
  A. Clinical Practice
  B. Advocacy
  C. Education
  D. Research
- The universal tasks of MS nursing are:
  A. Establishment of a therapeutic partnership
  B. Performance of a comprehensive assessment
  C. Formulation of a collaborative treatment plan
  D. Initiation, facilitation, and maintenance of a treatment regimen
  E. Evaluation of a treatment plan
- Domain: Clinical practice—Knowledge:
  A. Pathophysiology of disease:
    1. Immune dysfunction
    2. Nerve conduction

B. Definition, course, and classification
C. Epidemiology and distribution
D. Symptomatology
E. Diagnosis of multiple sclerosis:
    1. Presenting symptoms
    2. Prognostic indicators
    3. Diagnostic tests
F. Clinical practice—Knowledge and skills:
    1. Relapse management
    2. Disease modifying agents
    3. Symptoms and symptom management
    4. Psychosocial issues
G. Advocacy tasks
    1. Negotiate for the patient and family in the healthcare system
    2. Advocate self-care strategies
    3. Serve as a consultant
    4. Increase awareness of MS in the community
    5. Protect patient rights
    6. Examine practice outcomes
H. Advocacy requires knowledge and skills:
    1. Patient rights
    2. Ethical practice
    3. Negotiating the healthcare system
    4. Empowerment
    5. Public speaking
    6. Local and national health policy
    7. Disease expertise
■ Domain: Education:
A. Patient education:
    1. Knowledge of MS
    2. Nursing process and theory
    3. Principles of teaching/learning
B. Professional development:
    1. Role model
    2. Mentor
    3. Preceptor
    4. Public speaker
    5. Support group leader

6. Writer
7. Membership in professional organizations
■ Domain: Research:
A. Knowledge of research terminology and process
B. Protection of human subjects
C. Evidence-based practice.
D. Research tasks and skills:
1. Proper sample collection
2. Preparation and documentation
3. Communication skills
4. Research design, ethical principles
5. Drive to increase nursing body of knowledge

REFERENCE

Maloni, H. MSNICB, Toronto, Ontario, Canada. January 2002. Personal communication.

Chapter 3

Change Theory and Its Application in MS Nursing

Objectives:
Upon completion of this chapter, the learner will:

◆ Discuss the conceptual framework of change theory
◆ Describe its application in MS nursing

■ Systems theory is useful as a framework for viewing change since it provides a scheme for organizing information.

■ A systems theory model emphasizes unity and holism and seeks to avoid fragmented approaches.

■ The goal of a systems model is to provide a framework in which parts are connected and integrated.

■ Open systems freely exchange information and energy as they attempt to maintain a balanced state.

■ During change, the person of the change agent's system interacts with the patient's system to influence change and adaptation.

■ A change agent must be especially sensitive to feedback in order to determine how activities, ideas, and new programs are being accepted.

■ Change must be planned with respect for environmental systems and resources.

■ The change agent must be astute to recognize biased or erroneous sources of information so that undue system disruption does not take place.

■ One must consider the unique and highly personal values of each individual in order to initiate change.

■ Resistance can be minimized if the change agent keeps the systems open and dynamic.

■ The role of change agent is a challenging opportunity. Power is derived either from relationships or expertise or both. When the change agent advocates an innovation that is not satisfactory to the system, resistance can come into play.

■ These principles can be applied to patient and family education in terms of:

A. Adapting to new lifestyles related to MS

B. Changing roles and responsibilities

C. Learning and adopting complex protocols to manage MS

D. Adjusting to the dynamic nature of the disease

ADDITIONAL READING

Auger J. *Behavioral Systems and Nursing*. Englewood Cliffs, N.J.: Prentice Hall, 1976.

Lancaster J. *The Nurse as Change Agent*. St. Louis: CV Mosby Co., 1982.

Chapter 4

Multiple Sclerosis Nurses' Code of Ethics

A multiple sclerosis (MS) nurse has a professional moral obligation. The purpose of this obligation is to guide the MS nurse in the practice of multiple sclerosis nursing. This moral obligation is defined as performance of a morally good act, or rather, what ought to be done or should be done. The multiple sclerosis nurse provides care to promote the health and well-being of MS patients and families.

Ethical principles that guide the MS nurse are: beneficence, nonmaleficence, stewardship, autonomy, and justice.

Beneficence: Moral requirement to promote good
Nonmaleficence: Do no harm
Autonomy: Respect for self-determination
Stewardship: Preserve your own being
Justice: Fair and equitable determination distribution of resources and fair treatment for individuals and society

ANA Code of Ethics for Nurses

1. The nurse, in all professional relationships, practices with compassion and respect for the inherent dignity, worth, and uniqueness of every patient, unrestricted by considerations of social or economic status, personal attributes or the nature of the health problem.
2. The nurse's primary commitment is to the patient, whether an individual, family, group or community.
3. The nurse promotes, advocates for, and strives to protect the health, safety, and rights of the patient.

4. The nurse is responsible for and accountable for individual nursing practice and determines the appropriate delegation of tasks consistent with the nurse's obligation to provide optimum patient care.
5. The nurse owes the same duties to self as to others, including the responsibility to preserve integrity and safety, to maintain competence, and to continue personal and professional growth.
6. The nurse participates in establishing, maintaining, and improving healthcare environments and conditions of employment conducive to the provision of quality healthcare and consistent with the values of the profession through individual and collective action.
7. The nurse participates in the advancement of the profession through contributions to practice, education, administration, and knowledge development.
8. The nurse collaborates with other health professionals and the public in promoting community, national, and international efforts to meet health needs.
9. The profession of nursing, as represented by associations and their members, is responsible for articulating nursing values, for maintaining the integrity of the profession and its practices, and for shaping social policy.

(June 30, 2001 American Nurses Association)

■ Guiding principles of the MS nurse:
   A. Seeks what is good for patients and families.
   B. Recognizes that quality of life is defined by the person with MS.
   C. Recognizes and respects the patient's right to care regardless of age, race, gender, ethnicity, religion, lifestyle, sexual orientation, economic status, or level of disability.
   D. Recognizes the patient's right to MS specialist care.
   E. Promotes impartial treatment.
   F. Recognizes the patient's right to treatment and therapies, including experimental treatments.
   G. Recognizes the patient's right to access to MS drugs.
   H. Knows that patients have the right to be informed and understand advanced healthcare directives (living wills and durable

powers of attorney), concerning the right to receive resuscitation, refuse appropriate treatment, request do-not-resuscitate orders, or request the discontinuation of life support measures.

I. Is responsible for providing information to the MS patient and family in order to facilitate informed consent for all treatments and procedures.

J. Participates in research and is aware of the principles of informed consent, criteria for inclusion and exclusion in research protocols, and the right of the individual to withdraw from a protocol at any time.

K. Recognizes and maintains the patient's privacy, assuring confidentiality, except when there is a clear, serious, and immediate danger to the patient or others.

L. Has a moral obligation to offer access to care, cost containment, and quality care.

M. Affirms that MS patients have a right to be informed, without bias, coercion, or deception, about treatment options, potential effect, and adverse effects of treatments.

N. Supports the fact that MS patients have a right to refuse treatment, continuing to receive alternative care.

O. Recognizes that the MS patient has a right to review his medical record and the right to have information explained.

P. Requires participation of the MS patient in an ongoing partnership to develop an effective plan of care. This process considers diversity, individual autonomy, and responsibility.

Q. Practices competently, consulting and referring when indicated by professional judgment.

R. Takes appropriate action to protect patients from harm when endangered by incompetent or unethical clinical practice.

S. Promotes and supports improved practice through professionalism, education, certification, and nursing research.

T. Promotes local and national efforts to improve public education, legislation to ensure access to quality care, and long-term care initiatives that meet the health needs of MS patients and families.

REFERENCE

Maloni, H. MSNICB, Toronto, Ontario, Canada. January 2002. Personal communication.

Chapter 5

Epidemiology

Objectives:
Upon completion of this chapter, the learner will:

◆ Describe the difference between disease incidence and prevalence
◆ Provide an overview of the epidemiology of multiple sclerosis
◆ Discuss the implications of MS epidemiology in patient and family education

- Research into MS includes epidemiologic inquiries.
- Epidemiology is the study of the natural history of the disease.
- The *incidence* or *attack rate* is defined as the number of new cases of the disease beginning in a unit of time within a specified population. This is usually given as an annual incidence rate in cases per 100,000 per year. The date of onset of clinical symptoms decides the time of accession although, occasionally, the date of first diagnosis is used.
- *Prevalence* is easier to calculate than incidence because all cases are included regardless of disease duration. Nevertheless, accurate assessment of prevalence is still difficult because of the difficulty of full disease ascertainment.
- The *point prevalence rate* is more properly called a *ratio* and refers to the number of diagnoses within the community.
- The major clinical criteria in current use for MS are those by the Poser committee and a recent set of criteria that includes cases with monosymptomatic onset proposed by McDonald that strongly emphasizes MRI findings.
- Kurtzke classified MS prevalence rates into high, medium, and low risk groups. High-risk areas such as northern and central Europe,

Italy, the northern United States, Canada, southeastern Australia, New Zealand, and parts of the former Soviet Union are considered high risk, with rates greater than 30 per 100,000 populations.

- Medium-risk areas (prevalence between 5 and 29 per 100,000) include southern Europe, the southern United States, northern Australia, northernmost Scandinavia, much of the north Mediterranean basin, parts of the former Soviet Union, white South Africa, and possibly central South America. Low-risk areas (less than 5 per 100,000) include other areas of Africa and Asia, the Caribbean, Mexico, and possibly northern South America.

- As early as the 1920s it was recognized that the distribution of MS was not uniform. In general, people who reside in temperate climates in economically developed occidental countries tend to have a higher rate of MS.

- In the Northern Hemisphere, a diminishing north-south gradient has been well described.

- In the Southern Hemisphere, the reverse has been reported.

- There have been numerous reports of "clusters" in which several cases of MS have occurred at a similar point.

- Multiple sclerosis susceptibility has long been known to vary according to sex. Females are more susceptible than males in a ratio greater than 2:1.

- A review of the literature found that relatives (siblings, first-degree cousins, second-degree cousins) have an increased risk of MS susceptibility.

- Recent studies found a strong correlation for MS susceptibility in monozygotic twin pairs when compared with non-twin MS sibling pairs.

- The average age of onset is 10 to 59 years with the highest incidence between 20 and 40 years.

- The role of infectious agents as triggering factors has been proposed but there is no evidence to support this.

- Pregnant women have been followed through their pregnancies and to six months after delivery. There is a seven-fold decrease in exacerbations during pregnancy and a seven-fold increased risk during the six months after delivery.

- Several autoimmune diseases have been associated with multiple sclerosis. No data strongly link associations but anecdotal reports exist of relationships to diabetes mellitus, rheumatoid arthritis, myasthenia gravis, and bipolar illness.

■ Data are influenced by temporal differences as well as by differences in healthcare systems, neurologic expertise, and even by cultural practices.

■ Measures of disease frequency involve a numerator (cases), and a denominator (population at risk). Incidence and death rates refer to new cases and to deaths per unit time and population.

■ Prevalence rates refer to cases present at one time per unit populations.

■ Incidence and prevalence rates are derived from surveys of the disease within certain population; death rates come from published governmental sources.

■ There is a clear predilection for whites, but other racial groups share the geographic distributions of the whites although at lower levels.

■ Prevalence studies for migrants from high-risk to low-risk areas indicate the age of adolescence to be critical for risk retention, since those older than 15 years who migrate retain the MS risk of their birthplace. Those migrating before the age of 15 acquire the lower risk of their new residence.

■ Migration data support the idea that MS is ordinarily acquired in early adolescence with a lengthy "incubation" or latent period between disease onset and symptom onset. Susceptibility appears to extend to approximately age 45.

ADDITIONAL READING

Kurtzke JF, Wallin MT. "Epidemiology." In: Burks JS, Johnson KP, eds., *Multiple Sclerosis: Diagnosis, Medical Management, and Rehabilitation*. New York: Demos Medical Publishing, 2000; 49–71.

Kesselring J. "Epidemiology." In: Kesselring J, ed., *Multiple Sclerosis*. Cambridge: Cambridge University Press, 1997; 49–53.

Chapter 6

The Complete Neurologic Examination

Objectives:
Upon completion of this chapter, the learner will:

◆ Describe key components of a neurologic examination
◆ Discuss clinical implications of positive findings
◆ Cite the importance of patient and family education to explain the neuropathology of disease

■ Taking the history:
  A. The first and most important step in a focused assessment is gathering a detailed and accurate history in chronologic order.
  B. Family members or significant others may help contribute information.
  C. While taking the history, appraise the patient's conversational style. Is it coherent? Is the language fluent? Is the language appropriate for the level of education?
  D. Assess level of consciousness, orientation memory, intellectual status, and speech.
■ Mental status:
  A. The mental status assesses the following:
    1. Orientation to time: "What is the date today?"
    2. Registration: "Listen carefully. I am going to say three words and you repeat them to me after I stop."
    3. Naming: "What is this?" (Point to a pencil or pen.)
    4. Reading: "Please read this and do what it says." (Show the words on the stimulus form "Close your eyes.")
    5. The total score is a sum of each of the 11 evaluations. Each evaluation is scored with regard to the number of tasks per-

formed correctly. For example, if a patient is able to correctly recall only two of the three objects, a score of 2 is given. A mental status score of less than 20 points out of a maximum of 30 indicates a cognitive deficit.

■ Cranial nerves:

A. CNI—Olfactory nerve involves assessment of the sense of smell.

B. CNII—Optic nerve involves assessment of visual acuity and gross visual fields as well as an ophthalmosopic examination.

C. CNIII, IV, and VI are responsible for pupillary constriction elicited by shining a light into each eye. Each pupil should constrict directly and consensually (constriction of the opposite pupil). A pupillary difference (aniscoria) up to 20% may be pre-existing and normal. This nerve also innervates the extraocular muscles that affect lateral and vertical gaze and is tested with CN IV, which innervates the superior oblique muscle and aids in depression of the eye and looking downward, and CNVI, which innervates the lateral rectus muscle of the eye (abduction). Testing these three nerves involves testing the extraocular eye movements (nystagmus and isolated paralysis).

D. CNV, the trigeminal nerve, has both sensory and motor functions. Trigeminal neuralgia is a common problem in MS, and occurs when this nerve is affected.

E. CNVII has motor and sensory components. The motor portion innervates the muscles of the face and scalp; the sensory portion supplies the sense of taste on the anterior 2/3 of the tongue and sensation to the ear canal and behind the ear.

F. CNVIII is the acoustic nerve, which involves hearing and influences equilibrium.

G. CNIX supplies sensory sensation to the pharynx, tonsils, and posterior 2/3 of the tongue.

H. CNX is the vagus nerve; it is involved in the gag reflex and is tested with CNIX.

I. CNXI controls the movement of the sternocleidomastoid and trapezius muscles of the neck and shoulders.

J. CNXII is the motor nerve of the tongue.

TABLE 6.1   Summary of Cranial Nerve Function

Nerve	Function
I—Olfactory	Smell
II—Optic	Vision
III—Oculomotor	Eye movement, pupil contraction, accommodation, eyelid movement
IV—Trochlear	Up and out movement of eye
V—Trigeminal	Facial sensation, chewing
VI—Abducens	Lateral gaze
VII—Facial	Facial muscles, taste on anterior 2/3 of tongue, corneal reflex
VIII—Acoustic	Hearing
IX—Glosso-medulla	Taste, swallowing, gag reflex, cough
X—Vagus	Parasympathetic to organs, laryngeal muscles
XI—Accessory	Movement of head and shoulders
XII—Hypoglossal	Tongue muscles

- Motor assessment:
  A. Motor assessment techniques test muscle innervation by spinal nerves.
  B. Biceps involve elbow flexion and originate at C5 and C6.
  C. Triceps involve elbow extension and originate at C7, T1.
  D. Rectus abdominus involve trunk flexion and originate at T6-L1.
  E. Iliopsoas involve hip flexion and originate at L2 and L3.
  F. Quadriceps involve knee extension and originate at L2, L4.
  G. Biceps femoris involve knee flexion and originate at L5 and S2.
  H. Evaluation of arm drift is a sensitive test for weakness in the upper extremities.
  I. Other sensitive tests for extremity weakness include hand grasp, plantar flexion of the foot, and dorsiflexion of the foot.
  J. *Atrophy*—observe large muscle groups for symmetry and determine if their size is appropriate for the person's age.
  K. *Tone*—observe and test muscles for flaccidity, spasticity, or rigidity. Rigidity presents as stiffness regardless of the rate of passive movement. When an extremity is rigid, it "catches" during passive movement.
  L. Spasticity is dependent on the rate of movement. When the spastic extremity is moved slowly, the tone appears normal.

If the extremity is moved quickly, it "catches" and loses all resistance.

TABLE 6.2 Muscle Strength Grading (Oxford Scale)

0/5	No contraction
1/5	Visible/palpable muscle contraction but no movement
2/5	Movement with gravity eliminated
3/5	Movement against gravity only
4/5	Movement against gravity with some resistance
5/5	Movement against gravity with full resistance

- Sensory examination:
  A. Basic sensory examination consists of pain, light touch, proprioception, stereognosis, and vibration:
     1. *Proprioception* measures posterior column defects (position of toe—up or down, etc.)
     2. *Stereognosis* is dependent on touch and position sense (identification of a familiar object in one's hand).
     3. *Vibration sense* is tested by placing a vibrating tuning fork over the distal interphalangeal joint of a finger and the great toe.
- Cerebellum and gait:
  A. The cerebellum organizes and coordinates movements but does not control individual muscles. Smooth, coordinated movements depend on the normal functioning of the cerebellum. *Ataxia* describes disorganized, unsteady, or inaccurate movements. Tests include finger to nose, heel-knee-shin, the Romberg test, and gait assessment.
- Reflexes:
  A. The major deep tendon reflexes are:
     1. Achilles (S1, S2)
     2. Patellar (L3, L4)
     3. Biceps (C5, C6)
     4. Triceps reflexes (C7, C8)
     5. Grading is on a scale from 0–4+. Zero reflects no contraction (absent reflex), 1+ is diminished but present, 2+ is normal, 3+ is increased, 4+ is hyperactive with clonus.

6. Assymetric reflexes indicate neurologic (or muscular) dysfunction.

- Cerebellar disorders:
  A. *Ataxia*—awkwardness of posture and gait; tendency to fall to the same side as the cerebellar lesion; poor coordination of movement; overshooting the goal in reaching an object (*dysmetria*); inability to perform rapid alternating movements (*dysdiadochokinesia*), such as finger tapping; scanning speech due to awkward use of speech muscles, resulting in irregularly spaced sounds.
  B. Decreased tendon reflexes on the affected side.
  C. *Asthenia*—muscles tire more easily than normal.
  D. *Tremor*—usually an intention tremor (evident during purposeful movements).
  E. Nystagmus.
- Miscellaneous notes:
  A. The *left visual field* falls on the right half of each retina; the *superior visual field* falls on the inferior retina. The left visual field projects to the right side of the brain, and vice versa.
  B. The superior visual field projects below the calcarine fissure in the occipital lobe.
  C. Nystagmus is a repetitive, tremorlike oscillating movement of the eyes. The most common form is *horizontal jerk nystagmus*, in which the eyes repetitively move slowly toward one side and then quickly back. Vertical nystagmus is always abnormal, signifying a disorder in brainstem function.
  D. *Pendular nystagmus*, in which one eye moves at equal speeds in both directions, commonly is congenital.
  E. *Doll's Eye Phenomenon* occurs when the head is turned suddenly to one side. Normally, there is a tendency for the eyes to lag behind. This reflex is believed to be brainstem mediated, and any asymmetry or lack of response is believed to reflect significant brainstem dysfunction.

ADDITIONAL READING

Murray TA, Kelly NR, Jenkins S. The complete neurological examination: What every nurse practitioner should know. *Advance Nurse Practitioners* 10(July 2002); 7:24–30.

Chapter 7

Magnetic Resonance Imaging

Objectives:
Upon completion of this chapter, the learner will:

◆ Describe the role of MRI in the diagnosis and treatment of MS
◆ Discuss MRI in relation to disease modifying therapies
◆ Cite the use of MRI in MS research

■ Basic overview of MRI:
  A. Magnetic resonance imaging is commonly referred to as MRI.
  B. Unlike CAT (computed axial tomography) scans, MRI does not use X-rays to create pictures of the body.
  C. The technology uses a complicated array of physics, mathematics, and high-performance computing techniques.
  D. An MRI scanner consists of a very large and very strong, but harmless, magnet; the patient lies within the magnet's field.
  E. The scanner generates pictures by analyzing how water molecules react to electrical impulses in this strong magnetic environment.
  F. This involves radio frequency waves.

■ MRI principles:
  A. When a person lies in the magnetic field on an MR unit, protons align with the axis of the magnet.
  B. A radiofrequency pulse is transmitted, rotating the protons.
  C. When the pulse is turned off, the protons return to their previous states. Measurement of this activity is called T1 and T2.
  D. MS lesions have T1 and T2 relaxation properties because of free water associated with edema and inflammation and because of tissue destruction.

E. Pulse sequences used for MRI are known as spin-echo.

F. *Gadopentetate* (gadolinium) is a contrast agent to identify active MS lesions.

G. MS scans should include the entire brain, although MS lesions are most frequent in the periventricular region.

H. T1W or T1 *black holes* are subsets of chronic T2 lesions that appear hypointense on T1W images and have extensive tissue destruction.

I. It is likely that hypointense lesions on T1-weighted images represent the more disabling lesions and that these lesions correlate with persistent neurologic deficit in people with MS.

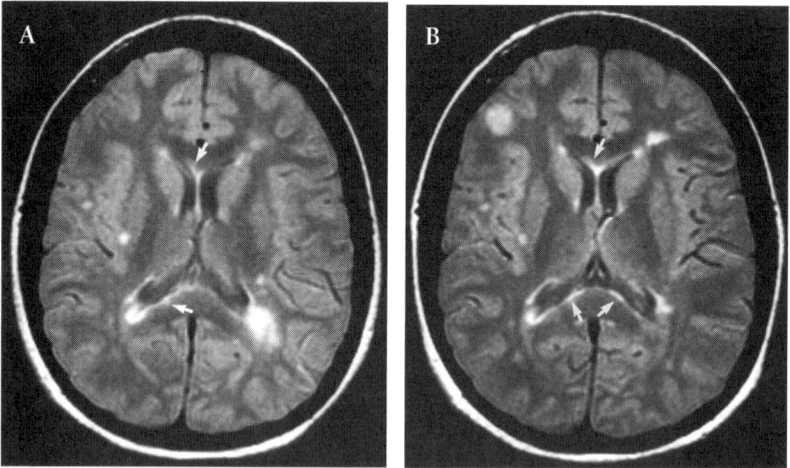

Lesions of the corpus callosum. Corpus callosum lesions (*arrows*) occur along the inner (deep) callosal surfaces and have irregular outer borders, which do not follow the expected contours of the nerve fibers. Axial (A and B) projections. Reprinted with permission. "Magnetic Resonance Imaging in the Diagnosis of Multiple Sclerosis, Elucidation of Disease Course, and Determining Prognosis," Simon JH. In: Burks JS and Johnson KP (eds.), *Multiple Sclerosis: Diagnosis, Medical Management, and Rehabilitation*, New York: Demos Medical Publishing, 2000.

■ Uses of MRI in MS:

A. The primary use of MRI in MS is to confirm the diagnosis and rule out other possible conditions.

B. MRI may also be able to predict the course of MS since research has shown that people who have MRI activity representing new MS lesions will continue to have MRI activity over subsequent months and years.

C. MRI may also be used to monitor the effectiveness of drugs in clinical trials.

D. MRI lesions may precede overt symptoms as seen in studies of the natural history of MS.

E. MRI has provided valuable insights into the course of the illness and has helped to identify new therapies that have at least a partial effect on disease activity.

F. Under the new diagnostic criteria proposed by McDonald, et al., T2 weighted lesions in the periventricular white matter, brain stem, and spinal cord, and Gd-enhancement on T1 imaging, along with hypointensities (black holes) on T1 images, support the diagnosis of MS.

- The evolution of the MS lesion:

A. Disruption of the blood-brain barrier with inflammation.

B. Gadolinium enhancement occurs at active sites.

C. This enhancement usually subsides in 3 to 6 weeks, leaving a "white spot" on the MRI image.

D. Sometimes these areas become larger and reinflamed with new disease activity, then once again subside.

E. Over time, repeated inflammation may cause extensive damage within the lesion, leaving what are known as black holes.

F. New MRI lesions can be "clinically silent." Several factors influence whether a lesion visible on MRI correlates with an overt clinical sign or symptom. These are:

1. Location of the lesion
2. Number of lesions
3. Severity of the damage

G. In the relapsing-remitting phase, a great deal of MRI activity occurs.

H. In the secondary-progressive phase, there are more symptoms and less MRI activity occurs; there are fewer acute inflamed lesions and more chronic, older lesions that reflect irreversible axonal damage and atrophy. MRI activity may fall off because there is less inflammatory activity.

I. The use of MRI in the diagnosis of MS and as a surrogate outcome measure has emerged as very important in diagnosing,

TABLE 7.1 Selected Features of MRI Measures*

Technique	Associated Pathology
T2 weighting	
New lesions	Inflammation
Enlarging T2 lesions	Increasing inflammation
T1 weighting	
Acute hypointense lesions ("black holes")	Edema associated with inflammation
Chronic hypointense lesions	Possible demyelination and axonal loss
Gadolinium-enhanced T1 weighting	Disruption of blood-brain barrier
Magnetization transfer	Changes in myelin
Magnetic resonance spectroscopy	
NAA peak	Axonal integrity
Lipid peak	Demyelination
Changes in brain volume	Brain atrophy

NAA=N-acetylaspartate
*From *MRI in the Management of MS,* page 3.

treating, and studying multiple sclerosis. It is likely that this technology will play a larger role in the long-term management of MS. Other technology, magnetization transfer MRI (MT) and magnetic resonance spectroscopy (MRS) have been applied to the evaluation of MS patients. MT changes may reflect changes in myelin although edema may also contribute to changes. MRS can detect changes in metabolites.

ADDITIONAL READING

Clanet M, Bates D, eds. *Imaging in Multiple Sclerosis.* MS Forum. Berlin: Schering AG, 1997.
Cook SD, ed. *The Multiple Sclerosis Handbook.* New York: Marcel Dekker, 2001.
McDonald et al. Recommended Diagnostic Criteria for MS. *Ann Neurol* 2001; 50:121–127.
Miller A, Johnson KP, Lublin F, Murray TJ, Whitaker JN, Wolinsky JS, eds. *MRI in the Management of MS.* Beechwood, Ohio: Current Therapeutics, Inc. 2002.

Chapter 8

Determining the Diagnosis and Prognosis of Multiple Sclerosis

Objectives:
Upon completion of this chapter, the learner will:

◆ Describe the pathophysiology of MS
◆ Describe common symptoms of MS
◆ Discuss the diagnostic process in MS
◆ Cite the common disease courses seen in MS
◆ Identify common laboratory tests used in the diagnostic process

Multiple sclerosis is a clinical diagnosis because there is no definitive laboratory test. It is common practice to perform a battery of pertinent investigations to exclude other conditions and to provide objective evidence that MS is the correct diagnosis. This also enables the neurologist to create a prognostic profile to guide therapeutic choices.

■ Pathophysiology of MS:
   A. The etiology of MS is not known.
   B. The most widely believed hypothesis is that it is a virus-induced autoimmune disease.
   C. A great deal of effort has gone into attempts to understand the immunology of MS using the animal model, experimental autoimmune encephalomyelitis (EAE).
   D. For normal nerve fibers, the myelin sheath has a uniform thickness and myelin segments between nodes of Ranvier (internodal segments) are of uniform length except near the end of each fiber, where internodes become progressively shorter.

E. The pathology of MS consists of lesions disseminated in location and of varying age. Lesions are present in both white and gray matter, but the gray matter lesions are less evident on casual inspection. Oligodendrocytes are damaged in this process.

F. Lesions range from acute plaques with active inflammatory infiltrates and macrophages loaded with lipid and myelin degeneration products to chronic, inactive, demyelinated scars.

G. Slowed conduction and conduction failure occurs in demyelinated fibers. Conduction failure is due to fiber fatigue or to an increase in body temperature or both.

H. Ongoing inflammation, demyelination, and scarring ultimately result in irreversible axonal damage and loss.

I. Acute MS lesions are characterized by T lymphohocytes, plasma cells, macrophages, and bare, demyelinated, or transected axons.

J. Brain atrophy in MS is widely recognized and represents a negative pathologic change. It may develop as an early measure of disease progression, and its slowing may be used as a measure of therapy efficacy in long-term management.

■ Demographics of MS:

A. Most patients are young women whose presenting symptoms are episodic neurologic problems that spontaneously improve.

B. The less common presentation is an older man or woman who has gradual development of neurologic deficits. Most often this takes the form of a progressive myelopathy.

C. 70 to 75% of patients with MS are female.

D. The only exception to this is in primary progressive MS, in which there is an equal ratio.

E. Most MS patients are Caucasian.

F. MS is rare among Africans, Asians, and Native Americans.

G. African Americans have levels of MS consistent with the mixing of the gene pool.

H. Asians are more likely to have spinal cord-optic nerve disease. This type of MS has an older age onset, fewer brain lesions on MRI, and more enhancing lesions in the spinal cord.

I. The average age of onset is 28 to 30 years.

J. Fewer than 1% have an onset before age 10; before age 16 1.2 to 6%.

- Prognostic factors in MS:
  A. Positive predictors in MS include:
  1. Younger age at onset
  2. Female sex
  3. Normal MRI at presentation
  4. Complete recovery from first relapse
  5. Low relapse rate
  6. Long interval to second relapse
  7. Low disability at 2 and 4 years
  B. Unfavorable predictors in MS include:
  1. Older age at onset
  2. Male sex
  3. High lesion load on MRI at presentation
  4. Lack of recovery from first relapse
  5. High relapse rate
  6. Early cerebellar involvement
  7. Short interval to second relapse
  8. Early development of mild disability
  9. Insidious motor onset
- Clinical profile of MS:
  A. Requires symptomatic disease over time, confirmed by objective evidence on neurologic examination. Symptomatic disease means neurologic worsening in the form of episodic attacks or slow progression.
  B. The most common presentations are:
  1. Sensory disturbance such as numbness, paresthesias, pain, or Lhermitte's sign (21–55% of patients):
     ✦ often begins in the limbs and migrates proximally, in
       ✧ tingling
       ✧ Lhermitte's
     ✦ neuritic pain
     ✦ diminished vibratory sensation
     ✦ impaired position sense
     ✦ "useless hand syndrome"
  2. Motor abnormalities:
     ✦ corticospinal (32–41%)
       ✧ heaviness, weakness, abnormal DTRs
       ✧ positive Babinski response

♢ spastic limb weakness
  3. Visual problems:
     ✦ brainstem
     ✦ eye movement abnormalities (diplopia nystagmus, INO)
     ✦ optic neuritis (in up to 25% of patients)
  4. Cerebellar gait ataxia limb ataxia tremor
C. Laboratory testing is used to help document that there are no
   alternative disorders to explain the neurologic picture and that
   there is a pattern of CNS lesion involvement consistent with
   MS, with no white matter involvement.
  1. Previous diagnostic criteria (Schumacher and Poser) have
     been supplemented by new criteria for a clinical isolated
     attack (CIS) to allow for an MRI supported diagnosis.
  2. The newer McDonald criteria, proposed in 2001:
     ✦ Developed by a large international committee funded by
       NMSS and MSIF to revise criteria to include new technology
     ✦ Preserves traditional diagnostic criteria of two attacks of
       disease separated in space and time
     ✦ Must be no better explanation
     ✦ Adds MRI, CSF, and EP criteria
     ✦ Three possible outcomes after work-up:
       ♢ Multiple Sclerosis
       ♢ Possible MS
       ♢ Not MS
     ✦ Monosymptomatic presentation:
       ♢ One attack
       ♢ One objective clinical lesion
       ♢ MRI evidence
     ✦ Primary progressive MS:
       ♢ Positive CSF and dissemination in space
       ♢ MRI evidence along with evoked potentials and CSF
       ♢ Continued progression over one year
     ✦ Although MRI is recognized as an invaluable tool, it is
       not appropriate to use it in isolation. Diagnosis should
       always be made in the clinical context.
     ✦ Paraclinical evidence along with MRI includes cerebro-
       spinal fluid with IgG oligoclonal bands or intrathecal
       IgG production.

◆ Evoked potential tests are used to document lesions disseminated in space to provide objective evidence to document subjective complaints or to confirm a pattern of CNS involvement consistent with MS. Nerve conduction is studied in the visual tracts, in the brainstem, and through the spinal cord (VEP, BAEP, and SEP).

■ Immunology of MS:
  A. The evidence for immune system involvement in MS is fairly clear while evidence that it is an autoimmune disease is more indirect.
  B. People with MS seem to have clear-cut abnormalities in immune function.
    1. Unusually high reactivity of immune system T-cells to proteins of myelin in the CNS (termed antigens since they can trigger immune responses)
    2. An over-representation of cells that enhance immune responses (T-helper cells).
    3. A relative under-representation of cells that suppress immune responses (suppressor T-cells)
    4. The presence of immune system cells in MS lesions in the brain, spinal cord, and optic nerves.
    5. Recently, the role of B-lymphocytes that are responsible for producing antibodies has been emphasized.
    6. "Direct" evidence that MS is an autoimmune disease is difficult to obtain in humans, but in the animal model (EAE), it is clear.
    7. Many studies during the latter part of the twentieth century increased our understanding of the immune system's reactivity to myelin in MS, including specificity immune responses to myelin antigens.

■ Etiology of MS:
  A. The genetic link in MS is borne out by the fact that:
    1. There is an increased susceptibility in certain families in which MS already occurs
    2. Some genetically isolated ethnic groups never develop MS (Hutterites in Canada; East European gypsies).
    3. The racial differences in MS prevalence are likely to be genetically based.

4. While genetics play a role in MS susceptibility, the nature of the link is both complex and largely unknown.
5. There is great interest in environmental triggering factors. Over the decades, there have been studies of retroviral (HTLV-1, HHV6, and canine distemper), and bacterial (chlamydia pneumoniae, et al.) triggers.
6. Evidence is anecdotal at this point, with no substantiation in research.

■ Clinical subtypes of MS (disease courses):
A. Primary progressive MS involves slow worsening from onset and is considered as a single attack. These patients may have to be observed over time; 15% of people with MS show this pattern.
B. Relapsing-remitting MS patients experience neurologic attacks with variable recovery but are clinically stable between attacks. Among this group are a minority of patients who will have minimal disease activity and little or no disability 25 years into their disease. These patients have benign or mild MS and may comprise 10 to 20% of those with MS.
C. Secondary progressive MS is the major progressive form of the disease and accounts for approximately 30% of all MS patients. These patients start with relapsing-remitting disease then slowly begin to worsen.
D. By 10 years, 50%, and by 20–15 years at least 80%, of untreated relapsing patients will become secondary progressive.
E. An additional term in the literature, *transitional MS*, refers to those patients who are evolving into the secondary progressive stage.
F. Some patients begin with no attacks and a progressive course, and later in their disease begin having exacerbations (progressive-relapsing).
G. Clinically isolated syndromes (CISs) are monoregional acute monophasic syndromes that encompass optic neuritis, transverse myelitis, isolated brainstem, or cerebellar syndromes. These patients have a high risk of MS, as confirmed by recent studies. MRI scans with T2 lesions predict a greater than 80% conversion to MS by 10 years.

■ Red flags in the diagnosis of MS:
A. One should be concerned about patients who:
1. Have not had any laboratory tests

2. Have normal neurologic examinations and normal laboratory studies
3. Have only peripheral nerve involvement
4. Have disease onset at a very early or very late age

ADDITIONAL READING

Coyle PK. "Diagnosis and Classification of Inflammatory Demyelinating Disorders." In: Burks JS, Johnson KP, eds., *Multiple Sclerosis: Diagnosis, Medical Management, and Rehabilitation.* New York: Demos Medical Publishing, 2000; 81–97.

Halper J. *The Nature of Multiple Sclerosis in Advanced Concepts in Multiple Sclerosis Nursing Care.* New York: Demos Medical Publishing, 2001; 1–25.

Martin R, Dhib-Jalbut S. "Immunology and Etiologic Concepts." In: Burks JS, Johnson KP, eds., *Multiple Sclerosis: Diagnosis, Medical Management, and Rehabilitation.* New York: Demos Medical Publishing, 2000; 141–165.

Chapter 9

The Immune System and Its Role in MS

Objectives:
Upon completion of this chapter, the learner will:

◆ Cite normal immune system activity
◆ Discuss abnormal immunology involved in MS
◆ Describe the rationale for immumodulating MS treatments

■ The immune system protects people from pathogens such as:
A. Bacteria
B. Viruses
C. Parasites
D. Fungi
E. Protects through:
  1. Innate immunity
  2. Adaptive immunity
■ The immune system comprises:
A. Innate immunity:
  1. Immunity to certain pathogens; this is common to all healthy individuals
  2. Does not require prior exposure to the pathogen
  3. Immediate destruction of some pathogens by phagocytic cells such as macrophage and neutrophils
B. Adaptive immunity:
  1. Requires exposure to pathogen to stimulate immune system response
  2. Cellular immunity
    ✦ Cytotoxic T-cells (CD 8)
    ✦ T_H1 cells (CD 4)

3. B lymphocytes
4. Antibodies
5. Activation of complement
C. Cells of the immune system begin life in the bone marrow as stem cells
D. T-cells are differentiated in the thymus
E. B-cells are differentiated in the bone marrow
F. These cells are activated in the lymphoid tissues where they are presented with antigen
G. B-cells recognize an antigen that is present outside of cells
H. T-cells detect antigens generated inside host cells
I. Both B-cells and T-cells must receive an additional signal in order to be activated
■ Humoral immunity is produced by:
A. Antibodies produced by B-cells
B. Antibodies work by
1. *Neutralization*—binding to pathogens and blocking the path to body cells
2. *Opsonization*—enabling phagocytic cells to recognize pathogens by coating the pathogen
3. Complement activation
■ Cellular immunity is produced by:
A. T-lymphocytes each having cell surface receptors:
1. Distinct from lymphocyte to lymphocyte
2. This enables lymphocytes to recognize a wide variety of antigens
B. Once a T-cell is activated by antigen presentation:
1. It proliferates in a process known as *clonal expansion*
2. Antigen-specific lymphocytes undergo apoptosis once the antigen is removed
3. Some antigen-specific lymphocytes persist and are the basis for immunologic memory
4. The cells that present antigen to T-cells are antigen-presenting cells
✦ dendritic cells
✦ macrophages
5. These cells display antigen protein particles on specialized cell surface molecules known as MHC.
6. Two classes of MHC molecules exist:

✦ MHC I

✦ MHC II

7. MHC I are recognized by cytotoxic T-cells (CD8).

8. MHC II are expressed on the surface of macrophages or B-cells and are recognized by T_H1 or T_H2 cells (CD4).

9. CD 4 Cell cytokine production:

✦ T_H1 cells activate macrophages and produce:

✧ interferon gamma

✧ TNF alpha

✧ TNF-beta

✧ IL-2

✦ T_H2 cells activate B-cells and produce:

✧ IL-4

✧ IL-5

✧ IL-10

✧ TGF-beta

■ Inappropriate immune response includes:

A. Allergy

B. Autoimmune disease

■ Allergy is the result of a specific IgE antibody to an innocuous antigen.

■ In autoimmune illness:

A. T-cells that recognize self-antigen are normally deleted.

B. The regulatory mechanisms that keep these cells in check are not working properly.

C. Without regulation, autoreactive T-cells can proliferate.

D. Molecular mimicry occurs:

1. Self-protein is structurally similar to non–self-antigen.

2. T-cells can recognize self-antigens if they are sufficiently similar to the non–self-antigen.

■ In multiple sclerosis:

A. T_H1 cells are stimulated in the periphery by presentation with antigen (i.e., a virus particle).

B. Once activated, they proliferate and release cytokines and met-alloproteinases that break down the extracellular matrix of the blood brain barrier (BBB).

C. Once in the CNS, T_H2 cells are presented with myelin protein that is similar to the antigen presented in the periphery.

   D. They then become reactivated, releasing the damaging
      cytokines interferon gamma, TNF-alpha, TNF-beta, and IL-2.
- Disease modifying treatments include:
   A. Immunomodulating and immunosuppressive agents that have
      an effect on some aspect of the immune response.
   B. With some agents, the effect is general, with others more specific.
   C. Interferon beta:
      1. Inhibits T-cell proliferation
      2. Inhibits synthesis of inflammatory cytokines (IFN-gamma,
         TNF-alpha)
      3. Downregulates expression of MHC class II molecules
         induced by IFN-gamma
      4. Reduces antigen presentation to T-cells
      5. Downregulates adhesion molecules and promotes BBB integrity
   D. Glatiramer acetate:
      1. Induces suppressor T-cells
      2. Is structurally similar to myelin basic protein. When
         GA-induced T-cells are presented to MBP in the CNS,
         they are stimulated to proliferate and release cytokines
         (TGF-beta, IL-4, IL-10)
   E. Immunosuppressants:
      1. *Cyclophosphamide* is a broad-spectrum immunosuppressant
      2. *Mitoxantrone* has a broad spectrum of immunosuppression
         with some B-cell suppression
      3. *Imuran* is a broad-spectrum immunosuppressant with milder
         effect and some B-cell suppression
      4. *Methotrexate* has little immunosuppression

ADDITIONAL READING

Costello K. *Immunology in MS*. Toronto, 2002. Personal communication.
Halper J, ed., *Advanced Concepts in Multiple Sclerosis Nursing Care*. New York: Demos Medical
   Publishing, 2001.
Halper J, Holland NJ, eds., *Comprehensive Nursing Care in Multiple Sclerosis*, 2nd Ed. New York:
   Demos Medical Publishing, 2002.
Paty DW, Ebers GC. *Multiple Sclerosis*. Philadelphia: FA Davis, 1998.

Chapter 10

Disease Altering Therapies

Objectives:
Upon completion of this chapter, the learner will:

◆ Discuss relapse management in multiple sclerosis
◆ Describe immunomodulation in relapsing forms of MS
◆ Cite management of worsening disease
◆ Describe strategies to promote adherence to complex protocols

■ Relapse management:
  A. A relapse is the appearance of a new symptom or the reappearance of a previous symptom of MS after the initial attack. A relapse cannot be related to an intercurrent infection or any other environmental factor and must last more than 24 hours.
  B. High-dose intravenous (or oral, depending on patient's place of residence) corticosteroids:
    1. Methylprednisolone
    2. Prednisone
    3. Dexamethasone
    4. ACTH (rarely used)
  C. No proof of benefit on relapse rates and progression
  D. Minimal evidence on optimal dose or regimen
  E. Protocols vary from country to country
■ Immunoregulators:
  A. Azathioprine (oral)
    1. No good double-blind, placebo-controlled studies but evidence suggests slight effect on disease activity
  B. Cyclophosphamide (IV or oral)
    1. Conflicting studies

2. High adverse effect profile
3. Many varying protocols
4. May be used for "rescue therapy"
C. Cyclosporine (IV)
1. Has been shown to have modest effect
2. High adverse effect profile
D. Methotrexate (oral)
1. Weekly low dose may help delay progression
2. Research demonstrates modest effect on upper extremity function
E. Mitoxantrone (IV)
1. Studied widely in Europe
2. Approved by FDA for worsening MS
3. Used in aggressive, relapsing MS and in patients with inadequate response to disease modifying agents
4. Has lifetime maximal dose
5. Potential for cardiotoxicity
F. Intravenous Immunoglobulin (IVIG)
1. Obtained from blood of healthy human donors
2. Still under investigation for use in MS with a double-blind placebo-controlled design
3. Some data on improved disability but no MRI data available as yet
4. Well tolerated
5. Very costly
■ Disease modifying therapy:
A. Therapies becoming available all over the world
B. Coverage varies greatly
C. In most countries, available for relapsing multiple sclerosis
D. Therapy initiation and ongoing adherence requires nursing services (documented in research)
E. Available therapies:
1. Interferon beta (1-b, 1-a)
2. Glatiramer acetate
3. Combination therapies
F. Interferon beta 1-b (Betaseron® or Betaferon®)
1. 8 MIU subcutaneously every other day
2. Requires reconstitution

TABLE 10-1   Disease Altering Therapies in MS

Drug and Dosage	Route of Administration	Side Effects and Nursing Implications
Interferon beta-1a Avonex 30 mcg IM q week	IM	Fever, chills, myalgia, asthenia, depression. Patient must be taught to reduce side effects with dose titration, injection in the evening, NSAIDS. Requires blood work (CBC, LFTs) at baseline, q 3 months then q 6 months thereafter. Needs reconstitution.
Interferon beta-1-a Rebif 22 mcg 3x q week 44 mcg 3x q week	SQ	Same as above for SE and blood work Site rotation required to prevent skin reaction Has prefilled syringes with auto injector
Interferon-beta-1b Betaseron 250 mcg qid every other day	SQ	Depression, injection site reaction, myalgia, fever, chills, menstrual irregularites. Same as above for SE management and blood work. Site rotation required. Has auto injector.
Glatiramer Acetate Copaxone 20 mg qd	SQ	Rare post-injection reaction with flushing, dyspnea, and anxiety. Injection site reaction Patient education re: side effects, need for site rotation, and reassurance about potential post-injection reaction. Has auto injector.
Azathioprine Imuran Dosage range from 50–200 mg	PO	Leukopenia lymphocytopenia. Patient must have CBC LFTs. Patient education important for monitoring blood values
Mitoxantrone (Novantrone) 12 mg/m^2 cumulative dose 140 mg/ m^2	IV	CBC, LFT's, echocardiogram or MUGA at baseline and regularly by Rx required. Side effects include myelosuppression, alopecia, secondar amenorrhea, cardiotoxicity. Patient education regarding SE and avoidance of infections. Need to adhere to follow up with blood work and cardiac monitoring.
Methotrexate 7–10 mg weekly	PO	Myelosuppression, vasculitis, nausea, vomiting. Patient education required to sustain adherence.
Cyclophosphamide with or without steroids or ACTH	IV	Myelosuppression, alopecia, secondary amenorrhea. Blood work required. Patient and family education to avoid infection.

Source: Adapted from Keegan & Noseworthy, 2002; Paty & Ebers, 1998.

3. Diluent available in prefilled syringe
4. Autojector for injection
5. Benefit in relapse rates and MRI
6. Preliminary data on cognition and depression
7. In secondary progressive MS, North American study was not statistically significant; in Europe, the results were positive
8. Side effect profile:
    ✦ flu-like syndrome
    ✦ skin reactions
    ✦ menstrual changes, abortifacient potential
    ✦ reports of depression (refuted in 2002, Feinstein et al.)
    ✦ neutralizing antibodies (NABs) 38%
    ✦ leukopenia
    ✦ elevated liver enzymes
    ✦ thrombocytopenia
9. Side effect management includes patient and family education in dose titration, timing of injections, NSAIDS, site rotation, management of depression.

G. Interferon beta 1-a (Avonex®)
1. 30 mcg (6MIU) weekly, requires reconstitution
2. Slows progression measured by EDSS in relapsing MS
3. Reduces relapses by 18%
4. Delays onset of CDMS by one year (monosymptomatic trial-CHAMPS)
5. No clear benefit in secondary progressive MS
6. Benefit in brain atrophy reported
7. Side-effects include:
    ✦ flu-like syndrome
    ✦ cautious use with seizures or depression
    ✦ abortifacient potential
    ✦ NABs 24%
    ✦ Elevated liver enzymes
8. Side effect management includes patient and family education in dose titration, timing of injections, NSAIDS, site rotation, management of depression

H. Interferon beta 1-a (Rebif®)
1. Two doses (22 mcg and 44 mcg) three times weekly subcutaneously

TABLE 10.2 Evidence-based Overview of Disease Altering Therapies

Drug	Manufacturere	Generic Name	Effect on Relapse Rate	Effect on Disease Progression as Measured by MRI	Effect on Disease Progression as Measured by Physical Disability
Avonex®	Biogen	Interferon beta-1a	18–21% reduction in 18–24 months	35–52% reduction in mean number of Gd-enhancing lesions in 12–24 months	37% reduced rate of accumulation of disability in relapsing-remitting MS
Betaseron®	Berlex	Interferon beta-1b	31% reduction in 24 months	Significant reductions in the burden of disease, in active treatment groups compared with placebo-treated patients, and a dose-effect was noted.	No significant progression of disability after 2 years; reduced clinical relapse rate by 34% after 2 years in relapsing-remitting MS
Rebif®	Serono	Interferon beta-1a	32% reduction in relapse rate at 24 months	84% reduction in Gd-enhancing lesions at 9 months	No significant progression of disability after 2 years
Copaxone®	Teva Neuroscience	Glatiramer acetate	33% reduction in relapse rate at 9 months	35% reduction in median number of Gd-enhancing lesions at 9 months; 50% reduction in neurodegenerative lesions ("black holes") within 9 months	Reduced clinical attack rate over 2 years; no statistical difference in the proportion of progression-free patients after 2years; 89% mean relapsing rate reduction after 8 years

2. Prefilled syringes with autojector (Rebiject®)
3. Dose-dependent decrease in relapse and MRI disease burden
4. Delayed onset of clinically definite MS by 9 months (ETOMS)
5. Side effects include:
   ✦ flu-like syndrome
   ✦ site reactions and rare necrosis
   ✦ menstrual irregularities
   ✦ leukopenia, elevated liver enzymes, thrombocytopenia
   ✦ NABs 23.8% low dose; 12.5% in high dose
   ✦ Possible depression, although this was refuted in a recent study
6. Side effect management includes patient and family education in dose titration, timing of injections, NSAIDS, site rotation, management of depression

I. Glatiramer acetate (Copaxone®) (combination of four amino acids
   1. 20 mg subcutaneously daily
   2. In prefilled syringe with autoinjector
   3. Sustained benefit in reduction of relapse rate
   4. Significant reduction of MRI lesion number and volume
   5. Being studied for primary progressive MS
   6. No statistical significance in oral form
   7. Side effects include:
      ✦ injection site reactions and pain
      ✦ rare systemic reaction (chest pain, dyspnea, and anxiety—post-injection reaction)
      ✦ arthralgia and nausea

J. Common problems with disease modifying agents (DMAs):
   1. Spasticity
      ✦ Commonly seen with interferon therapy
      ✦ May occur on initiation of therapy or prior to treatment
      ✦ Differential diagnosis between interferon-induced spasticty or spasticity associated with relapse or infection is necessary
      ✦ Assess for other contributing factors
      ✦ Administer anti-spasticity medications

✦ Consider dose adjustment of interferons until problem is managed
2. Laboratory abnormalities
    ✦ No known significant abnormalities with glatiramer acetate
    ✦ In interferon therapy, the most common abnormalities are leukopenia, neutropenia, and raised liver aminotransferase values (e.g., serum glutamic oxaloacetic [SGTOT] and serum glutamic pyruvic transaminase [SGPT])
3. Managing laboratory abnormalities:
    ✦ Monitor lab values regularly following initiation of treatment
    ✦ Inform physician of abnormal values
    ✦ Consider dose adjustment and/or discontinuation of treatment if abnormalities persist
K. Combination therapy
    1. Several studies of small sample size have shown benefit of combination therapy.
    2. Some of the combinations studied include Betaseron® and azathioprine; Betaseron® and Mitoxantrone®; Avonex®, and Cytoxan®; Avonex® and Cytoxan®; Avonex® and azathioprine; Copaxone® and Betaseron®; Avonex® and Copaxone®.
L. Initiation of therapy
    1. Regardless of who makes the decision, it is imperative that the nurse educate the patient and family on:
        ✦ all available treatments
        ✦ efficacy and side effects
        ✦ self-care activities
        ✦ the importance of adherence
M. The Psycho-Educational approach
    1. Requires that the patient and family become actively involved in goal setting, realistic expectations, and the process itself
N. Patient and family education require that:
    1. Information is provided in a clear and concise manner.
    2. There is a relaxed and non-distracting learning environment.

3. A variety of educational tools are utilized.
4. Reinforcement is provided regularly.
5. Education should not be initiated immediately after diagnosis.
6. Hope can be instilled along with realistic expectations.
7. Patients must be motivated to learn; if they are not ready, education should be delayed.
8. Outcomes of education:
   ✦ Patient should be able to:
      ✧ describe rationale of therapy
      ✧ correctly reconstitute and administer medication
      ✧ manage side effects
      ✧ identify and use resources to obtain further information
9. Promoting adherence:
   ✦ establish a trusting relationship
   ✦ consistent and clear education
   ✦ advocate for access to treatment
   ✦ reinforcement of the multidisciplinary team
   ✦ ongoing patient and family contact

ADDITIONAL READING

Burk JS, Johnson KP, eds., *Multiple Sclerosis: Diagnosis, Medical Treatment, Rehabilitation*. New York: Demos Medical Publishing, 2001.

Halper J, ed., *Advanced Concepts in Multiple Sclerosis Nursing Care*. New York: Demos Medical Publishing, 2001.

Halper J, Holland NJ, eds., *Comprehensive Nursing Care in Multiple Sclerosis*. New York: Demos Medical Publishing, 2002.

MS Nurse Specialist Committee. Multiple sclerosis: Key issues in nursing care. Adherence, cognition, quality of life. Columbia, Md. Medicalliance, 1997.

MS Nurse Specialist Committee. Best practices in nursing care: Disease management, pharmacological treatment, nursing research. Columbia, Md. Medicalliance, 1998.

Van den Noort S, Holland NJ, eds., *Multiple Sclerosis in Clinical Practice*. New York: Demos Medical Publishing, 1999.

Chapter 11

The Symptom Chain in Multiple Sclerosis

Objectives:
Upon completion of this chapter, the learner will:

◆ Describe the most common symptoms of MS
◆ Cite effective management strategies of MS symptoms
◆ Discuss the nurse's role in symptomatic management

■ Multiple sclerosis is a complex and dynamic disease.
  A. It has a wide variety of disease patterns.
  B. Signs and symptoms vary from person to person or within the individual.
  C. Fluctuation is based on circumstances.
  D. Many symptoms have a cascade effect on functioning.
  E. Careful management can improve quality of life.
  F. Ongoing, poorly managed symptomatic problems can be devastating.

■ The key to management is knowledge and skills:
  A. Symptoms have to be recognized, understood, and discussed with the healthcare team by the patient and family.
  B. Management should be individualized and flexible in light of the dynamic nature of MS.

■ Common symptoms of multiple sclerosis:
  A. Fatigue
  B. Depression
  C. Focal muscle weakness
  D. Visual changes
  E. Bowel/bladder/sexual dysfunction
  F. Gait problems/spasticity
  G. Paresthesias

TABLE 11.1 Commonly Used Pharmacologic Interventions

Generic Name	Brand Name	Usage in MS
Alprostadil	Prostin VR	Erectile dysfunction
Alprostadil	Muse	Erectile dysfunction
Amantadine		Fatigue
Amitriptyline	Elavil	Pain (paresthesias)
Baclofen		Spasticity
Bisacodyl	Dulcolax	Constipation
Carbamazepine	Tegretol	Pain (trigeminal neuralgia)
Ciprofloxacin	Cipro	Urinary tract infections
Clonazepam	Klonopin (US); Rivotril (Can)	Tremor; pain; spasticity
Desmopressin	DDAVP nasal spray	Urinary frequency
Dexamethasone	Decadron	Acute exacerbations
Diazepam	Valium	Spasticity (muscle spasms)
Docusate	Colace	Constipation
Docusate mini enema	Therevac Plus (US)	Constipation
Fluoxetine	Prozac	Depression; fatigue
Gabapentin	Neurontin	Pain
Glycerin	Sani-Supp suppository (US)	Constipation
Imipramine	Tofranil	Bladder dysfunction; pain
Magnesium hydroxide	Phillips' Milk of Magnesia	Constipation
Meclizine	Antivert (US); Bonamine (Can)	Nausea; vomiting; dizziness
Methenamine	Hiprex, Mandelamine (US); Hip-rex, Mandelamine (Can)	Urinary tract infections (preventative)
Methylprednisolone	Depo-Medrol	Acute exacerbations
Mineral oil		Constipation
Modafinil	Provigil	Fatigue
Nitrofurantoin	Macrodantin	Urinary tract infections
Norfloxacin	Noroxin	Urinary tract infections
Oxybutynin	Ditropan	Bladder dysfunction
Oxybutynin (extended release formula)	Ditropan XL	Bladder dysfunction
Papaverine		Erectile dysfunction
Paroxetine	Paxil	Depression

continued on next page

TABLE 11.1 Commonly Used Pharmacologic Interventions (continued)

Generic Name	Brand Name	Usage in MS
Pemoline	Cylert	Fatigue
Phenazopyridine	Pyridium	Urinary tract infections (symptom relief)
Phenytoin	Dilantin	Pain (dyesthesias)
Prednisone	Deltasone	Acute exacerbations
Propantheline bromide	Pro-Banthine	Bladder dysfunction
Psyllium hydrophilic mucilloid	Metamucil	Constipation
Sertraline	Zoloft	Depression
Sildenafil	Viagra	Erectile dysfunction
Sodium phosphate	Fleet Enema	Constipation
Sulfamethoxazole	Bactrim; Septra	Urinary tract infections
Tizanidine	Zanaflex	Spasticity
Tolterodine	Detrol (US)	Bladder dysfunction
Venlafaxine	Effexor	Depression

■ Less-common symptoms of multiple sclerosis:
  A. Dysarthria, scanning speech, dysphagia
  B. Lhermitte's sign
  C. Neuritic pain
  D. Vertigo/ataxia
  E. Cognitive dysfunction
  F. Tremor/incoordination
■ Rare symptoms of multiple sclerosis:
  A. Decreased hearing
  B. Convulsions
  C. Tinnitus
  D. Mental disturbance
  E. Paralysis
■ Fatigue
  A. May be directly due to MS
  B. Other causes: depression, deconditioning, medications, concommitant medical conditions (thyroid dysfunction, cardiovascular disease), sleep disturbance
  C. The most common cause of MS-related disability

D. Can be managed with a wide variety of strategies
E. Evaluation:
  1. Assess for impending exacerbation
  2. Screen for infection
  3. Question about environmental factors (heat, humidity)
  4. Ascertain medications, dosages, and time of dosing
  5. Assess sleep habits
  6. Question about other symptoms (pain, spasticity, bowel or bladder dysfunction)
  7. Assess mood
  8. Evaluate activity level and physical fitness
E. Management:
  1. Instruct in effective energy expenditure
  2. Encourage the use of appropriate use of assistive devices (scooters, walkers, wheelchairs, transfer equipment)
  3. Encourage the use of air conditioning and other cooling techniques
  4. Encourage the treatment of mood disorders
  5. Encourage the initiation of symptom management—pain, spasticity, bowel, bladder dysfunction
  6. Advocate for the treatment of medical conditions causing fatigue
  7. Improve sleep hygiene
  8. Medications used to manage MS-related fatigue:
    ✦ CNS stimulants (methylphenidate)
    ✦ aminopyridines (currently being studied in research)
    ✦ amantidine (SE: headache, dizziness, rash)
    ✦ modafinil (SE: headache, tachycardia, palpitations, contraindicated in LMVP)
    ✦ pemoline (liver cautions)
    ✦ SSRI antidepressants
    ✦ unique antidepressants—buprioprion (Wellbutrin®) (SE: seizure risk)
   9. Initiate appropriate conditioning programs
  10. Reassess patient on a regular basis
■ Pain
  A. Pain is complex; it is a sensory phenomenon
  B. Pain inadequately defined, identified, or measured by an observer

C. Pain is an individual, learned, social, and cultural response

D. A common myth in MS is there "is no pain"

E. Both acute and chronic pain can be related to MS:
   1. Acute pain
      + trigeminal neuralgia
      + tonic spasms
      + lightning-like extremity pain
      + painful Lhermitte's sign
      + optic neuritis and retrobulbar pain
   2. Chronic pain with insidious onset
      + dysesthetic extremity pain
      + bandlike pain in torso or extremities
      + back pain with radicolopathy
      + headache

F. Trigeminal neuralgia probably arises from transmission of nerve impulses in areas of demyelination.
   1. Treatment consists of IV or oral steroids in the acute phase.
   2. In the chronic phase, anticonvulsants such as carbamazepine and gabapentin are used.

G. Painful tonic spasms may or may not be related to spasticity. Simple flexor spasms may be related to movement or noxious stimuli. Treatment consists of antispasticity medications and anticonvulsants.

H. Less common is the painful tetanic posturing of an arm or leg, usually on one side of the body. Treatment consists of carbamazepine, clonazepam, tizanidine, and baclofen.

I. Lightning-like extremity pain can be treated with carbamazepine, gabapentin, and phenytoin.

J. Lhermitte's sign responds to the above medications and also to tricyclic antidepressant medications.

K. Headache has been reported to be causally related to demyelinating lesions. Treatment generally proceeds along the lines of headache without MS. When associated with a relapse, treatment with steroids may cause resolution of headache.

L. Optic neuritis is due to inflammation and demyelination occurring in and around pain-sensitive meninges surrounding the optic nerve. Steroid treatment usually brings resolution of the pain.

M. Commonly used medications:
1. *Phenytoin*—best in dysesthetic pain
2. *Gabapentin*—useful in dysesthetic and paroxysmal pain; better SE profile than phenytoin
3. *Carbamazepine*—effective in pain of paroxysmal onset; e.g., trigeminal neuralgia
4. *Clonazepam*—effective in bandlike sensations
5. *Baclofen*—useful in trigeminal neuralgia
6. *Misoprostol*—contraindicated in pregnancy
7. *Lamotrigine*—limited use due to interactions and adverse events
8. *Tramadol*—helpful in a variety of nonrefractory pain syndromes
9. *Tizanidine*—useful adjunct in chronic pain syndrome

■ Spasticity
A. 60% of people with MS have corticospinal tract involvement with some degree of spasticity
B. Accentuation of DTR and clonus occurs, with exaggeration of flexor reflexes
C. Spasms and stiffness are common in the quadriceps, hamstrings, and gastrocnemious muscles
D. May be heightened during an exacerbation, with underlying infection, and with noxious stimuli
E. Physical therapy techniques are designed to:
1. Avoid secondary complications such as decubitus ulcers
2. Prevent or treat contractures
3. Reduce muscle hypertonia by stretching spastic muscles and by application of warm or cold packs
4. Improve patient's posture
5. Develop and improve useful automatic movements and thus promote maximal function
6. Assist the patient to learn more coordinated movements
7. Supply supportive aids such as walkers, wheelchairs, crutches, orthoses, and special shoes
F. Screening for noxious stimuli will promote prompt treatment and reduction of spasticity.
G. Medications for spasticity may be sedating and excessive doses may result in weakness

    1. Baclofen

    2. Tizanidine

    3. Clonazepam

    4. Diazepam

  H. Intrathecal baclofen (ITB)

    1. Surgically implanted pump for intrathecal baclofen delivery
- no systemic side effects
- expensive
- requires surgery
- reserved for patients in whom other interventions are unsuccessful

■ Tremor, incoordination, and weakness

  A. Most difficult problems to modify in MS

  B. Pharmacologic regimens tend to be sedating and have limited benefit

  C. Physical and occupational therapy may provide patient with education and assistive devices, but do not correct the underlying problem

■ Dysarthria

  A. Normal speech consists of five systems working together smoothly and rapidly:

    1. *Respiration*—using the diaphragm to fill the lungs fully

    2. *Phonation*—using the vocal cords and air flow

    3. *Resonance*—raising and lowering the soft palate

    4. *Articulation*—making quick, precise movements of the lips, tongue, mandible, and soft palate

    5. *Prosody*—combing all elements for natural flow of speech

  B. Speech impairment has long been considered a principal symptom of MS.

  C. Three types of dysarthria are associated with MS:

    1. Spastic

    2. Ataxic

    3. Mixed dysarthria

  D. In MS, a mixed spastic-ataxic dysarthria is typical.

  E. There are no medications for the speech problem itself. Treatment consists of management of spasticity and tremor along with speech and language therapy (SLT)

F. When to refer to SLT:
 1. Are problematic speech and voice characteristics detracting from the message being communicated?
 2. Are speech and voice adequate for daily communication?
 3. Are speech, voice, and communication problems interfering with the patient's quality of life?
 4. Are speech, voice, and communication problems perceived as troublesome by the patient and family?

■ Dysphagia
 A. Normal swallowing involves intricate and rapid coordination of sensory and motor activity in the oral cavity, pharynx, and esophagus.
 B. Normal oromotor control for swallowing involves lip closure, facial tone and musculature, rotary lateral jaw motion, and pharyngeal swallow.
 C. Due to MS, the following may occur:
 1. A delay in triggering the pharyngeal swallow
 2. Difficulty managing thin liquids
 3. Problems in the oromotor control phase
 4. Reduced tongue coordination
 5. Possible esophageal involvement
 6. Food aversions due to altered taste sensations
 D. Assessment includes a careful history (pneumonia, difficulty with liquids and solids, aspiration or choking while eating).
 E. Optimal management includes referral to a speech/language pathologist familiar with MS and its related problems.
 F. Videofluoroscopic examination or modified barium swallow (MBS) may identify the patient's swallowing pathology. The resulting report should include a description of the patient's physiologic or anatomic swallowing abnormalies; any symptoms associated with the problem; results of any treatment attempted; and recommendations for treatment and dietary intake.
 G. Treatment procedures involve:
 1. Changing the individual's head or body posture
 2. Controlling the volume and speed of eating
 3. Educating patients and families about voluntary swallowing maneuvers

   4. Educating patients and families about fatigue and dysphagia
      with advice to rest during long meals and/or to eat more
      often for a shorter time
■ Sexuality and intimacy
   A. Primary sexual dysfunction occurs as a result of MS-related
      physiologic changes in the CNS that directly impact sexual
      feelings and/or response
   B. Symptoms:
      1. Decreased or absent libido
      2. Altered genital sensations
      3. Decreased frequency, intensity of orgasms
      4. Erectile dysfunction
      5. Decreased vaginal lubrication/clitoral engorgement
      6. Decreased vaginal muscle tone
   C. Management:
      1. Men—pharmacologic management of erectile dysfunction
         (injections, Viagra®)
      2. Women—medications (Viagra®, lubrication, body mapping
         assessment)
   D. Secondary sexual dysfunction occurs as a result of MS-related
      physical changes and treatments that indirectly affect sexual
      feelings and/or response
   E. Etiology
      1. Bladder or bowel dysfunction
      2. Fatigue
      3. Non-genital sensory paresthesias
      4. Spasticity
      5. Cognitive impairment
      6. Tremor, pain
   F. Management:
      1. Treat underlying symptoms
      2. Work with symptoms
         ✦ positioning comfortably
         ✦ using spasticity to maintain body contact
      3. Review and adjust medications
   G. Tertiary sexual function is due to psychological, social, and
      cultural issues that interfere with sexual feelings and/or
      response. Origins are:

1. Clinical depression
2. Grief
3. Changes in self image and body image
4. Family and social role changes
5. Anger, guilt, depression
6. Spousal burden as caregiver

H. Management:
   1. Counseling of patient and family
   2. Grief work
   3. Acknowledgment and treatment of intermittent problems
   4. Culturally sensitive interventions with appropriate support

I. The nurse's role in working with sexuality and intimacy problems:
   1. Evaluate personal attitudes, values, and beliefs
   2. Assess personal knowledge
   3. Sustain comfort level in patient/partner interaction

J. Some leading questions are:
   1. Has anything interfered with your ability to maintain closeness?
   2. How do you feel about being a man/woman?
   3. How has MS changed, if at all, your ability to function sexually?

K. Some sexual assessment tools are:
   1. The Sexual Health Assessment Framework (Szasz, 1989)
      + sexual knowledge
      + sexual self-view
      + sexual activity
      + sexual interest and behavior
      + sexual response
   2. PLISSIT Model

L. Working with sexuality and intimacy
   1. Open, nonjudgmental atmosphere
   2. Ensure privacy
   3. Encourage open questions
   4. Normalize and validate concerns
   5. Part of the review of systems
   6. Offer resources and reassurance

■ Cognition
   A. The causes of cognitive changes may be divided into primary and secondary effects of the disease.

B. Primary effects:
1. The nerve cells themselves
2. Lesions are multifocal and vary from person to person in distribution
3. This may be explained by cerebral demyelination and axonal damage
C. Secondary effects:
1. Depression
2. Anxiety
3. Stress
4. Fatigue
D. Frequency, severity, and nature of cognitive changes
1. Estimates range from 45 to 65% of people with MS having changes
2. Only 10% suffer from severe impairment
3. No correlation between disease course, disease severity, or length of time since diagnosis
4. In most cases, cognitive dysfunction is characterized by selective impairment of some functions with relative preservation of others
5. Cognitive functions thought to be affected:
   ✦ memory (working memory and secondary memory)
   ✦ abstract reasoning and problem solving
   ✦ attention and concentration (especially sustained or complex attention)
   ✦ speed of information processing
   ✦ verbal fluency
E. What is seen clinically?
1. Inability to think
2. Inability to remember
3. Inability to reason logically
F. The nurse role is:
1. Establish a relationship with patients and families
2. Facilitate communication
3. Observe and assess
4. Initiate referrals
5. Promote coping strategies
6. Monitor for safety

G. Impact of cognitive impairment:
  1. Role strain
     ✦ social roles
     ✦ work roles
H. Evaluation of cognitive impairment
  1. Informal evaluation
     ✦ tool selection
     ✦ nursing assessment
  2. Formal neuropsychological evaluation by neuropsychologists
     ✦ patient selection
     ✦ patient support
  3. Cognitive rehabilitation (mediocre results)
  4. Potential benefit from disease modifying agents
  5. Nursing interventions
     ✦ recognizing and acknowledging deficits
     ✦ accurate report of evaluation results
     ✦ patient and family support
■ Depression
  A. Disorders of mood and affect
     1. Major depression (subsyndromal depression, suicide is 7.5% greater than general population)
     2. Bipolar affective disorder
     3. Euphoria
     4. Pathologic laughing and crying (mood swings)
  B. Major depression
     1. Lifetime in approximately 50% with MS
     2. Point prevalence approximately 14%
     3. Increased compared to other neurologic disorders
  C. Possible causes and contributors to depression in MS:
     1. Disease activity (especially exacerbations)
     2. Neuropathologic changes in areas of the brain concerned with affective states
     3. Neuroendocrine or psychoneuroimmunologic changes
     4. Reaction to altered life circumstances
     5. Medication side effects
  D. Assessment of depression should be done on a regular basis.
  E. Tools = CESD, Zung Depression Scale, or Beck Depression Inventory (preferred via consensus)

F. Treatment of depression:
  1. Counseling and emotional support, psychotherapy
  2. Pharmacologic management
     ✦ tricyclic antidepressants
     ✦ mood stabilizing agents (Depakote®, lithium carbonate)
     ✦ SSRIs (fluoxetine, sertraline, paroxetine, venlafexine)
     ✦ St. John's Wort (complementary or alternative medication [CAM])
     ✦ support and therapeutic groups
■ Nursing care
  A. Empowers patients with knowledge and skills development
  B. Assists patients to make informed decisions
  C. Establishes an interdependent trusting relationship
  D. Encourages patients to share expectations, desires, and values
  E. Contributes to health-related quality of life (HRQOL) in MS
     1. HRQOL is a state of complete well-being and not merely the absence of disease/infirmity.
     2. It is degree of satisfaction with perceived present life circumstances.
     3. It is the perception of the impact of the disease both subjectively and objectively.
     4. It is a multidimensional construct emphasizing perceptions.
     5. MS has an effect on QOL through its array of symptomatology. Disease disruption ranges from mild to severe and may vary over time according to disease course and available supports.
     6. Specific issues related to MSQOL:
        ✦ alterations in social environment
        ✦ role reversals in family relationships
        ✦ social and emotional isolation
        ✦ misinterpretation of symptoms by others
        ✦ restricted range of opportunities
        ✦ alterations in body image
        ✦ impact upon intimate relationships
     7. Roles of the nurse in MSQOL:
        ✦ facilitating adjustment to MS
        ✦ establishing a comfortable relationship
        ✦ providing education and information
        ✦ supporting, emphathizing, and "cheerleading"

- ✦ communicating, collaborating, and creating
- ✦ assisting with adjustment during the post-diagnosis period and throughout lifetime
- ✦ empowering patients through self-determination and self-advocacy
- ✦ simply being there when needed
8. Strategies to maintain MSQOL:
  - ✦ Encompass the patient's ability to:
    - ✧ adapt
    - ✧ communicate
    - ✧ socialize
    - ✧ be productive
  - ✦ Adapt
    - ✧ responding to change
    - ✧ identifying and evaluating options
    - ✧ setting, resetting, and achieving flexible goals
  - ✦ Ability to communicate
    - ✧ developing and maintaining satisfying relationships
    - ✧ determining whether changes are needed in relationships
    - ✧ seeking supportive and reciprocal relationships
  - ✦ Ability to be productive
    - ✧ contributing to home work, school, or volunteer activities
    - ✧ feeling that one's opinions matter to others
    - ✧ participating in meaningful activities
9. Significance when patients are cognitively impaired:
  - ✦ importance of selecting the right style of education
  - ✦ memory aids to help at home
  - ✦ frequent follow-up
  - ✦ reinforcement of actual expectations
  - ✦ ongoing education of patient/family
  - ✦ working with the MS team

ADDITIONAL READING

Burks JS, Johnson KP. *Multiple Sclerosis: Diagnosis, Medical Management, and Rehabilitation.* New York: Demos Medical Publishing, 2001.

Halper J, ed., *Advanced Concepts in Multiple Sclerosis Nursing Care.* New York: Demos Medical Publishing, 2001.

Halper J, Holland NJ, eds., *Comprehensive Nursing Care in Multiple Sclerosis.* New York: Demos Medical Publishing, 2002.

Holland NJ, Halper J, eds., *Multiple Sclerosis: A Self-Care Guide to Wellness.* Washington, DC: PVA, 1998.

Lowden, D. Sexuality and intimacy. Toronto, Canada. January 2002. Personal communication.

Chapter 12

The Multiple Sclerosis
Care Team

Objectives:
Upon completion of this chapter, the learner will:

◆ Describe the key participants in the MS team
◆ Discuss the role of the nurse in MS rehabilitation
◆ Describe the role(s) of rehabilitation in MS

■ When is rehabilitation provided in multiple sclerosis?
   A. *Acute*—during and following exacerbations
   B. *Episodic*—when functional status changes occur
   C. *Maintenance*—ongoing strategies to sustain function and
      prevent injury and trauma
■ Rehabilitation sites
   A. Inpatient facilities
   B. Outpatient care
   C. Home care
   D. Community support programs
   E. Fitness programs
■ The MS rehabilitation team
   A. Patient/family
   B. Physical therapists
   C. Occupational therapists
   D. Speech and language therapists
   E. Neurologists
   F. Physiatrists
   G. Nurses
   H. Psychologists
   I. Neuropsychologists

J. Social workers
K. Clergy
L. Case managers
M. Community assistants (advocates, NMSS, organizations that support the disabled)
■ Adapting to change
A. Functional status
B. Assistive devices
C. Educational needs
D. Environmental modifications
E. Vocational rehabilitation
F. Economic concerns
G. Long-term planning
■ Supporting the family through the rehabilitation period
A. Counseling
B. Education
C. Emotional support
D. Ongoing communication
E. Advocacy
■ Principles of neurorehabilitation in MS:
A. Should be dynamic, flexible, and creative
B. Issues such as patient and family adherence, cognitive impairment and its effect on learning, and quality of life should be considered when planning and implementing new strategies and employing new techniques
C. Neurorehabilitation in MS requires a team approach with collaboration among the team, the patient, and the family
D. Considerations in neurorehabilitation include:
   1. Insurance coverage
   2. Family support
   3. Patient's social, cultural, and economic environment
   4. Ability to carry out treatment plan
■ Supporting transitions in MS
A. Acknowledge the problems
B. Refer the patient to appropriate resources
C. Assist with access to adequate services
D. Coach, partner, reassure
E. Re-evaluate on a regular basis

- Empowerment
  A. Empower with:
  1. Modeling
  2. Tools
  3. Modifications
  4. Education
  5. Support
  6. Encouragement of decision making and self-efficacy

ADDITIONAL READING

Kennedy P. "Interfacing with Rehabilitation Services." In: Halper J, Holland NJ, eds., *Comprehensive Nursing Care in Multiple Sclerosis*. New York: Demos Medical Publishing, 2002; 147–174.

Schapiro RT. *Symptom Management in Multiple Sclerosis*. Demos Medical Publishing, 2000.

Chapter 13

Bladder Dysfunction

Objectives:
Upon completion of this chapter, the learner will:

◆ Describe the anatomy and physiology of the urinary tract
◆ Describe the neurologic innervation of the urinary tract
◆ Describe diagnostic procedures used in the management of urinary dysfunction in MS
◆ Describe prevention and management of urinary dysfunction and MS
◆ Describe nursing interventions in bladder management in MS

Approximately 80% of patients with MS experience significant bladder dysfunction at some point in the course of disease. Bladder dysfunction causes alterations in personal, social, and vocational activities along with sleep disruption, embarrassment, dependency, and isolation. Nursing plays a major role in the assessment and treatment of bladder dysfunction and is designed to help the individual with MS achieve a predictable and effective elimination plan and to minimize complications.

■ Treatment goals
  A. Maintain renal function
  B. Keep patient dry
  C. Establish normal voiding patterns
  D. Reduce symptoms and improve quality of life
  E. Motivate patient to adhere to treatment
■ Normal urinary function
  A. The kidneys of an adult female produce 100 to 125 ml per hour.

B. Males produce closer to 150 ml per hour.

C. The actual rate depends on fluid intake, position, and kidney function.

D. Kidneys produce urine more efficiently in the supine position; thus, diuresis may become a problem for patients with heart or lung problems.

E. Ureters are thin-walled muscular tubes that move urine from the kidneys to the bladder.

F. Closure of the ureters during bladder contraction is accomplished by contraction of the trigone area during voiding.

G. The main function of the urinary bladder is to store and expel urine.

H. The bladder is a hollow muscular organ that is supported by loose connective tissue. The trigone and lower portion of the base of the bladder rest upon the anterior vaginal wall in women. The wall of the bladder consists of inner mucous membrane with a cell lining and underlying lamina propria; a layer of smoother muscle, the detrusor; and an outer layer of connective tissue.

I. The urethra has an internal and external sphincter mechanism. The interior sphincter has three components (urethral mucosa, periurethral connective tissue, and periurethral vascular plexus). Each is responsible for one-third of the urethral closure pressure. The internal sphincter is composed of small muscle bundles and is not under voluntary control. The external sphincter is under voluntary control.

J. The bladder is innervated by sympathetic fibers from the hypogastric nerve at T10 through L2 and parasympathetic fibers from the pelvic nerve at S2 through S4.

K. As the bladder fills with urine, its fundus rises into the lower abdominal cavity.

L. To initiate voiding, the urethra relaxes first, then the bladder contracts and expels the urine through the relaxed sphincter. These functions occur automatically.

M. Average bladder capacity for an adult is 300 to 500 ml. The initial urge to void occurs when approximately 200 ml has accumulated. Contractions of the bladder are inhibited by the nervous system until 300 ml has been collected. An individual

can sense bladder fullness and can initiate or postpone emptying as convenient.

N. Normally a person voids 4 to 6 times during a 24-hour period,
depending on fluid intake, type, and amount.

■ Problems occurring in MS

A. Bladder dysfunction in MS is primarily associated with
demyelination in the spinal cord, the pontine cerebellar
micturition control areas, or other CNS points in between.

B. Interruption of the spinal cord pathways may result in excessive detrusor contractions, involuntary sphincter relaxation or
contraction, or detrusor areflexia with urinary retention.

C. Bladder dysfunction, or neurogenic bladder, may produce:

1. *Urinary urgency*—a strong need to urinate that cannot be
controlled or postponed

2. *Urinary frequency*—the need to urinate more often than
every 2 to 3 hours

3. *Urinary hesitancy*—difficulty initiating the flow or urine

4. *Nocturia*—waking up more than once during the night to
urinate

5. *Incontinence*—losing control of urine

6. *Incomplete emptying*—feeling that some urine is left in the
bladder after urinating

7. *Urinary tract infections (UTIs)*—resulting in classic symptoms of
burning or pain upon urination. This may result in a tempo-
rary worsening of MS symptoms or may be the first sign that a
person is experiencing a change in usual bladder function.

D. The presence of one or more of these symptoms is suggestive
of a neurogenic bladder.

E. The three common types of bladder dysfunction are the result of:

1. Hypercontractility of the detrusor muscle

2. Inability of the sphincter to relax and open, or detrusor
areflexia

3. Incoordination of the detrusor and sphincter activity: detrusor-
sphincter dyssynergia (DSD)

F. In summary, bladder dysfunction in MS can result in failure to
store urine, failure to empty urine, or combined dysfunction.

G. Similar symptoms may be present in all three types of bladder
dysfunction.

■ Assessment of bladder dysfunction
  A. Evaluation of patient's chief concern
  B. Voiding pattern, daytime and nighttime
  C. History of incontinent episodes
  D. Urinary patterns and symptoms—urgency, frequency, inconti-
     nence, hesitancy, hematuria, use of protective pads, dysuria, UTIs
  E. Medical history—surgery, number of full-term pregnancies,
     gynecologic problems
  F. Current medications
  G. Evaluation of post-void residual via straight catheterization or
     bladder ultrasound.
     1. In straight catheterization patient drinks two 8-ounce glasses
        of water prior to assessment.
        ✦ patient voids and output is measured.
        ✦ patient is catheterized for post-void residual urine.
        ✦ greater than 100 ml, the patient requires instruction in
          self-catheterization
        ✦ frequency of self-catheterization depends on amount of
          urine remaining in the bladder after voiding.
          ✧ if there is 100 ml in the bladder, can be done once daily
          ✧ if more than 200 ml, twice daily
        ✦ If residual is less than 60 ml, patient is prescribed med-
          ications to control/reduce bladder spasms and promote
          more efficient bladder storage of urine
  H. Bladder ultrasound
     1. Full bladder is scanned for total volume of urine in bladder
     2. Patient then voids
     3. Bladder is rescanned to determine post-void residual
  I. Follow-up is the same as above.
  J. With intermittent self-catherization in the failure-to-empty
     bladder, the addition of anticholinergic or antimuscarinic med-
     ication may be considered to reduce patient's symptoms
     despite fully emptying of the bladder.
■ Additional studies:
  A. Kidney and bladder ultrasound can yield information about
     structural abnormalities causing symptoms
  B. Intravenous pyelogram (IVP) can outline the ureters and is also
     a test of kidney function.

C. Urodynamic studies clarify the function of the muscles of the lower urinary tract. Complete urodynamic testing includes uroflowmetry, the quantitative and qualitative analysis of urinary stream. It is the measurement of the rate of urination and force of the bladder's expulsive ability.

D. Pressure flow parameters in the study include bladder pressure, rectal pressure, differential pressure, urethral pressure, flow rate, volume, and electromyogram (EMG) sphincter activity.

E. Both needle and surface EMG and CMG (filling cystometrogram) are helpful in diagnosing detrusor-sphincter dyssynergia.

■ Bladder management interventions:

A. Bladder training consists of education, scheduled voiding, and positive reinforcement. This requires that the participant resist or inhibit the sensation of urgency to postpone voiding, and urinate according to a timetable rather than according to the urge to void.

B. Bladder training may also involve tactics to allow the bladder to hold a greater volume:

1. Drinking an adequate amount of fluid at one sitting will generally result in an urge to void within the retraining time frame.
2. Avoiding fluids with caffeine, artificial sweeteners, and alcohol will reduce bladder irritability.
3. Protective pads may absorb involuntary urine outflow.
4. Male external catheters may help do the same.
5. Medications that are beneficial for failure to store and DSD include:
   ✦ anticholinergics (oxybutynin)
   ✦ antimuscarinics (tolterodine tartrate, hyoscyamine sulfate)
   ✦ tricyclic antidepressants (imipramine)
   ✦ antidiuretic hormone analog (desmopressin acetate), particularly for nocturia

C. Crede method is contraindicated because of the potential to create increased pressure and damage the upper tract.

D. Intermittent self-catheterization (ISC)

1. Allows an individual to empty the bladder at regular intervals, thereby reducing the risk of UTI, structural damage, and other distressing bladder symptoms.
2. This technique has been widely supported in the literature. It uses a clean technique. Teaching guides are available

E. An indwelling catheter may be needed for either short- or long-term use and allows for continual drainage by gravity.
   1. Its use is suggested for those individuals who cannot be managed with ISC and/or medications, or who have chronic decubiti and cannot perform ISC.
   2. Long-term use of indwelling catheters is a significant source of bacteruria and UTI. Management varies but the usual practice is to change the catheter after a minimum of 30 days or prn. If the patient has a symptomatic UTI, the entire system must be changed and a urine culture obtained.
   3. A person with MS may still experience urinary incontinence with an indwelling catheter. In this instance, the indication is not to increase the size of the catheter or balloon, but rather to use anticholinergic/antimuscarinic medications to decrease urinary tract spasticity.
■ Surgical interventions:
A. Suprapubic catheters are sometimes an alternative to long-term urethral catheters. These may be helpful in male patients and in women who have developed severe urethral irritation secondary to an indwelling Foley catheter.
B. Sphincterectomy may be recommended for very disabled male patients who experience intractable hesitancy and retention. Anticholinergic medications and an external condom catheter can be combined to manage bladder activity.
C. Some female patients with small-capacity bladder may benefit from a laparoscopic procedure that includes bladder augmentation with a continent diversion. Patients then can catheterize a stoma at the navel or abdomen.
D. Diversion procedures including cystostomy or transurethral resection, which provides a clear passageway for the urine to flow freely. This procedure is used only rarely.

ADDITIONAL READING

Dierich M. "Bladder Dysfunction." In: Burks JS, Johnson KP, eds., *Multiple Sclerosis: Diagnosis, Medical Management, and Rehabilitation*. New York: Demos Medical Publishing, 2000; 433–452.
Frenette J, Harris C, et al. "Symptom Management." In: Halper J, ed., *Advanced Concepts in Multiple Sclerosis Nursing Care*. New York: Demos Medical Publishing, 2001; 175–184.
Holland N. *Bladder and Bowel Management. Multiple Sclerosis; A Self-Care Guide to Wellness.* Washington, D.C.: PVA, 1998; 5–1.
Namey M. "Management of Elimination Dysfunction." In: Halper J, Holland N, eds., *Comprehensive Nursing Care in Multiple Sclerosis*. New York: Demos Medical Publishing, 2002; 53–65.

Chapter 14

Bowel Elimination and Continence

Objectives:
Upon completion of this chapter, the learner will identify:

- ◆ The common pathophysiology of upper motor neuron bowel, lower motor neuron bowel, uninhibited neurogenic bowel, and motor paralytic bowel as seen in MS
- ◆ Goals for establishing bowel control with MS
- ◆ Common nursing interventions in managing a neurogenic bowel
- ◆ A comprehensive care plan for gastrointestinal complications
- ◆ The long-term implications of neurogenic bowel dysfunction

Altered bowel function may occur whenever the central nervous system (CNS) has been impaired. When disease or disability results in altered bowel control, incontinence may become as devastating a problem as the disease itself. Control of incontinence and prevention of constipation and diarrhea are possible through an effective bowel program, which requires a knowledge of normal and altered bowel physiology as well as an in-depth assessment of bowel function.

- ■ Normal bowel anatomy and physiology
  - A. The lower bowel acts under voluntary control to store and eliminate feces.
  - B. Inability to store fecal matter causes problems with involuntary bowel or incontinence.
  - C. Inability to eliminate causes constipation.
  - D. The bowel consists of three separate parts: the ileum, the cecum, and the colon.

E. The *ileum* is approximately the last third of the small intestine.
   1. It is approximately 12 feet long and extends from the jejunum to the ileocecal opening.
   2. Almost all absorption and digestion is accomplished in the small intestine.
   3. The small intestine absorbs water and sodium and secretes mucus, potassium, and bicarbonate for stool formation.
F. The *cecum* is 6 cm in length and lies below the terminal ileum, forming the first part of the large intestine.
G. The *colon* is the division of the large intestine that extends from the cecum to the rectum.
   1. In the colon, fluids and electrolytes are reabsorbed and feces are stored so that defecation can occur at an acceptable time.
   2. Defecation is affected by peristalsis, anorectal sensory awareness, anal sphincter function, and abdominal muscle function and strength.
H. The *rectum* is the 12 cm segment of the large bowel between the sigmoid colon and the anal canal. As a rule, it does not contain feces except during defecation.
I. The *anal canal* comprises the last 3 cm of the digestive tubes. Striated muscle in the anal canal and pelvic floor provides support to the rectal wall and anus, thus maintaining continence.

■ Neurogenic bowel
A. Constipation:
   1. Neurogenic bowel results from the interruption of neural pathways that supply the rectum, external sphincter, and accessory muscles involved in defecation.
   2. Nerve impulses that are disrupted may impede cerebral recognition of anal contents and the need to empty stool at a desired or planned time.
   3. Slowed transit may result in constipation.
   4. Weakened abdominal muscles may make bearing down very difficult.
   5. Decreased activity related to altered mobility, fatigue, or a sedentary lifestyle may contribute to slow bowel function.
   6. Constipation has been defined as less than or equal to two bowel movements per week; or the need for stimulation, the use of laxatives, enemas, or suppositories more than once a week.

7. Constipation has also been characterized by hard, dry stool, causing straining or painful defecation and resulting in a delay of passage of food residue.

8. Medications contributing to constipation may include
   + analgesics
   + anticholinergics
   + anticonvulsants
   + antidepressants
   + diuretics
   + psychotherapeutics
   + iron
   + opiates
   + muscle relaxants

9. Other neurologic factors that contribute to neurogenic bowel conditions:
   + lack of exercise
   + inadequate fluid intake
   + inadequate dietary fiber
   + effects of medication

10. Diarrhea may result from gastrointestinal influenza, dietary irritants, and gastrointestinal disorders.

B. Diarrhea or involuntary bowel:

1. Diarrhea (loose, liquid stools) and frequent discharge of fluid fecal matter may be secondary to
   + fecal impaction
   + diet or irritating foods
   + inflammation or irritation of the bowel
   + stress, anxiety
   + medications
   + overuse of laxatives or stool softeners
   + dietary intolerance of milk products, chocolate

2. Diarrhea may be accompanied by urgency, cramping, abdominal pain, increased bowel sounds, or increased volume of stools.

3. In MS, involuntary bowel or fecal incontinence is the result of interruption in the neural pathways and impaired cortical awareness of the urge to defecate.
   + characterized by urgency and involuntary stools

  ✦ defecation is sudden with or without urgency
  ✦ patient may also experience partial or total sensory loss in
    the perineum and rectum
■ Assessment and management of bowel function/dysfunction
  A. Questions to ask include the use of medications that influence
     bowel activity, such as diuretics, antacids, nonsteroidal
     anti-inflammatory agents, anticholinergics, antidepressants,
     antibiotics, laxatives, and enemas.
     1. Presence or absence of the awareness of the need to defecate.
     2. Frequency and quality of stool including color and consistency.
     3. Fluid and dietary history should include fluid intake, daily
        intake of fiber, and type of food or snacks eaten.
     4. Objective assessment of the abdomen should include aus-
        cultation, palpation, and percussion.
     5. Assessment should include patient's functional ability to
        ambulate and transfer, the use of assistive devices, the ability
        to remove clothing, and the accessibility of toilet facilities.
  B. Interventions to manage bowel dysfunction:
     1. Goals of bowel training program include:
        ✦ normalizing stool consistency
        ✦ establishing a regular pattern for defecation
        ✦ stimulating rectal emptying on a routine basis
        ✦ avoiding complications of diarrhea, constipation, or
          incontinence
        ✦ improving the patient's quality of life
  C. Constipation should be first treated with nonpharmacologic
     interventions:
     1. Increased fluid intake (1 to 2 quarts daily), fiber, exercise.
     2. Education and support are equally important.
     3. Establish a regular pattern of bowel elimination.
     4. Use the gastrocolic reflex.
     5. Sit in an upright position with feet on the floor.
     6. The program may take 3 to 4 weeks or longer.
     7. The use of stool softeners or bulk formers with fluids and
        fiber may help.
     8. Oral stimulants provide a chemical stimulation and a
        localized mechanical stimulation and lubrication to
        promote elimination of stool.

9. Glycerin suppositories provide lubrication for passage of stool.
10. Dulcolax® suppositories and Therevac® mini enemas contain medications that stimulate strong, involuntary, wavelike movement that facilitates the elimination of stool.
11. Regular use of enemas should be avoided to minimize the risk of dependency.
12. Fecal impaction is a complication of chronic constipation: manual disimpaction or soap suds enemas are the options for immediate treatment, but long-term management with the above is the appropriate option.
13. An episode of fecal impaction is an indication for the need for an aggressive bowel program.

D. Fecal incontinence:
1. Adequate bulk and fiber is important for maintenance of stool consistency. Patients should be instructed to avoid overly spicy and gas-forming foods.
2. Planned times for bowel evacuation and the use of suppositories to stimulate rectal emptying allows for more bowel control.
3. Establishing a routine eliminates involuntary bowel accidents.
4. Encourage the patient to sit on a toilet or commode for 25 to 30 minutes after consuming a hot beverage.
5. The following strategies may help:
   ✦ sit comfortably on the toilet and try to "bear down"
   ✦ rocking back and forth and massaging the abdomen can promote bowel activity
   ✦ if the bowels do not move within 10 minutes, leave the bathroom and try again later when another "urge" is present

E. Expected outcomes of bowel management:
1. Predictable, regular bowel evacuation.
2. Decrease in episodes of constipation or involuntary bowel.
3. Formed stool.
4. Avoidance of prescription drugs, strong laxatives, or enemas.
5. Patient and family awareness of the elements of bowel management.
6. Patient and family awareness of early signs of bowel dysfunction.

ADDITIONAL READING

Holland NJ. "Bladder and Bowel Management." In: Holland N, Halper J, eds., *Multiple Sclerosis: A Self-Care Guide to Wellness.* Washington, D.C.: PVA, 1998; 5–1.

Namey M, Halper J. "Bowel Disturbance." In: Burks JS, Johnson KP, eds., *Multiple Sclerosis: Diagnosis, Medical Management, and Rehabilitation.* New York: Demos Medical Publishing, 2000; 453–459.

Namey, M. "Elimination Dysfunction in Multiple Sclerosis." In: Halper J, Holland N, eds., *Comprehensive Nursing Care in Multiple Sclerosis.* New York: Demos Medical Publishing, 2002; 64–69.

Chapter 15

The Nurse's Role in Advanced Multiple Sclerosis

Objectives:
Upon completion of this chapter, the learner will:

♦ Describe key issues of concern in advanced MS
♦ Discuss nursing implications in progressive disease
♦ Cite specific strategies in avoiding complications of this advanced condition

■ Advanced MS
  A. A small percentage (5%) of people with MS become severely disabled
  B. Caregivers are faced with ongoing tasks and special needs in this population
  C. The nurse is challenged as both a caregiver and educator of the patient, family, and responsible others in the patient's life
■ Nutrition
  A. General nutrition
    1. A well-balanced diet is important throughout one's lifetime—sick or well.
    2. Good nutrition is characterized by a well-developed body with ideal weight, healthy hair and skin, and mental alertness.
    3. RDA recommendation by the U.S. Department of Agriculture are guidelines for health professionals and patients.
    4. Recommendations include servings in bread and cereal group, vegetable and fruit groups, limiting fat intake, and adequate intake of water and fluids.
    5. There is no conclusive evidence that any nutritional therapy affects the course of MS.

6. The nurse is in an excellent position to educate patients and families about nutrition.
B. MS factors that can affect nutrition
1. Tremor, weakness, paralysis, and dysphagia can interfere with nutrition.
2. Fatigue and depression may alter nutritional status.
C. Managing nutritional problems:
1. Patient's weight should be monitored.
2. A swallowing evaluation should be recommended when indicated.
3. A registered dietitian can determine caloric needs based on activity level.
4. A person with skin breakdown will need increased calories and protein to promote healing.
5. Feeding techniques and education may be required in a person with dysphagia.
6. Referrals to home health programs to relieve the caregiver may be necessary.
7. Meals-on-wheels or food stamps may be helpful.
8. Those with decreased energy may precook or microwave meals.
9. Small, frequent feedings may be recommended.
10. Adaptive equipment such as weighted utensils, elongated straws, and modified dishes may be helpful.
11. Nutritional supplements may ensure adequate intake in patients with fatigue.
12. Fluid intake in advanced MS:
   ✦ minimum of 8 glasses needed daily (1500–2000 ml/24 hours)
   ✦ UTIs can be reduced with acidification and hydration
   ✦ fluids can be obtained through gelatin and other desserts
   ✦ supplemental tube feedings may be necessary
■ Urinary tract infections (UTIs)
A. UTIs pose a serious threat in advanced MS.
B. Urinary drainage may be accomplished through spontaneous voiding, IC, or indwelling catheter.
C. While IC is the preferred artificial way of emptying the bladder, indwelling catheters are a reality in advanced disease.

    D. Attention must be given to keep tubing and drainage bags as clean as possible.

    E. Catheters should be changed regularly.

    F. Patients must be monitored for signs and symptoms of UTI (fever, U/A, C&S, increased spasticity, etc.)

    G. Treatment of UTIs (symptomatic vs. colonized) should be initiated promptly.

- Spasticity

    A. Management is a challenge because of intercurrent symptoms such as fatigue and weakness.

    B. Medications consist of baclofen, tizanidine, dantrolene, diazepam, and gabapentin.

    C. Stretching, positioning, and ROM are important to maintain muscle length and tone.

    D. Blocks and surgical techniques may be beneficial.

    E. The advent of intrathecal delivery of baclofen is a breakthrough in the management of intractable spasticity.

    F. Pump maintenance and dose titration are relatively simple.

- Skin care

    A. Prevention of skin breakdown is essential.

    B. Braden and Norton Scales have been validated in MS.

    C. Braces or splints may cause friction or pressure.

    D. Maintenance of desired weight is important.

    E. Nursing activities include:

        1. Identification of predisposing factors

        2. Patient and family education

        3. Use of appropriate assistive devices for transfers

        4. Regular skin inspection

        5. Maintenance of bowel and bladder continence

        6. Adequate personal hygiene

        7. Adequate nutrition and fluid intake

- Personal care

    A. Formal and informal caregivers may be required.

    B. Respite care is important to prevent burnout.

    C. Alternative long-term solutions may need to be explored.

    D. Day treatment programs may relieve caregiver burden.

- Family needs

    A. Advanced directives should be discussed.

B. Life planning should be encouraged.
C. Counseling and education are essential to support family needs.
D. Community agencies are important assets at this time.
E. Opportunities to communicate fears and concerns are important.

ADDITIONAL READING

Harris C. "Prevention of Complications in the Severely Disabled." In: Halper J, Holland N, eds., *Comprehensive Nursing Care in Multiple Sclerosis.* New York: Demos Medical Publishing, 2002; 93–122.
Halper J. *Nursing Care in Advanced MS.* Toronto: January, 2002. Personal communication.

Chapter 16

Psychosocial Implications

Objectives:
Upon completion of this chapter, the learner will:

◆ Describe initial reactions to the diagnosis of MS
◆ Discuss the emotional impact of worsening disease
◆ Cite therapeutic nursing interventions in support of patients
  and their families

■ Reactions to the diagnosis:
  A. Shock
  B. Disbelief
  C. Denial
  D. Anger
  E. Depression
  F. Despair
  G. Curiosity
  H. Information seeking
  I. Needing to affiliate with others
  J. Wanting to be cured
  K. Facing the reality of change
■ Emerging issues in MS:
  A. There is a greater understanding of MS with an emphasis on
     early intervention.
  B. People with MS are faced with adapting to unpredictable
     change.
  C. There are issues of abuse and neglect, divorce and separation,
     altered body image.
  D. The challenge is to sustain a high level of support.

- Long-term implications for MS nurses:
  A. Need to assess family resources
  B. Need for environmental adaptations
  C. Need for life planning
  D. Impact on future relationships
  E. Need for advocacy to access programs and services
  F. Sustaining realistic hope
- Employment issues:
  A. Reasonable accommodations
  B. Vocational rehabilitation
  C. Telecommuting
  D. Cognitive implications
  E. Educational concerns
- Impact on the family:
  A. Alterations in roles and responsibilities
  B. Child-bearing and child-rearing concerns
  C. Changing lifestyles and economic circumstances
  D. Grief work balanced with hope
- How information helps children:
  A. Provides reassurance
  B. Allays fears
  C. Gives them a vocabulary
  D. Reduces secrecy
  E. Promotes trust
  F. Gives symptoms a name
- Managing change in MS:
  A. Education about the disease throughout a lifetime
  B. Counseling and support groups
  C. Crisis intervention
  D. Long-term planning/life planning
  E. Being flexible
  F. Finding hope
  G. Seeking wellness

ADDITIONAL READING
La Rocca NG, Kalb RC. "Psychosocial Issues in Multiple Sclerosis." In: Halper J, Holland NJ, eds., *Comprehensive Nursing Care in Multiple Sclerosis*. New York: Demos Medical Publishing, 2002; 93–122.

Chapter 17

Financial and Vocational Concerns

Objectives:
Upon completion of this chapter, the learner will:

◆ Describe the provisions of private and public health insurance plans
◆ Describe factors that promote and hinder employment of persons with MS
◆ Describe the provisions of vocational rehabilitation assistance programs

■ Cost of living with MS
   A. Reasons for determining costs include:
      1. Guide the selection of treatment modalities
      2. Guide the allocation of research dollars
      3. Locate hidden costs
   B. Costs of MS over a lifetime vary from country to country; they may exceed a minimum of $1,000,000 in lost wages, medical costs, and inestimable family expenses
■ Health insurance programs
   A. United States private health insurance plans
      1. Traditional indemnity plan
      2. Managed care plans
      3. Health maintenance organizations
      4. Preferred provider organizations
   B. U.S. governmental plans
      1. Supplemental Security Income (SSI)
      2. Social Security Disability (SSD)
      3. Civilian Health and Medical Program of the VA

    4. Medicare
    5. Medicaid
  C. Canadian healthcare system
    1. All people receive healthcare coverage
    2. Most people with MS must be assessed by MS specialists for DMAs (not in all provinces)
  D. Canadian governmental disability plans
    1. Canadian Pension Plan Disability Program (CPP)

- Importance of employment
  A. Promotes feelings of personal worth and self-esteem
  B. Contributes to one's identity
  C. Source of respect from others
  D. Provides monetary income
  E. Frequent source of health insurance

- Factors that influence unemployment
  A. Demographics
    1. Age
    2. Education
    3. Female sex
    4. Laborer status
  B. Psychosocial
    1. Cognition
    2. Depression
    3. Motivation
  C. Physical
    1. Gait and mobility
    2. Fatigue
    3. Visual disturbance
    4. Bladder/bowel function
  D. Environment
    1. Accessibility
    2. High temperature
    3. Transportation

- Factors that enhance employment and work
  A. Personal attributes
  B. Psychological and social services
  C. Vocational services

- Employment protection

A. The Americans with Disabilities Act (ADA)
  1. Prohibits discrimination on basis of disability
  2. Requires reasonable accommodation
  3. Public transportation running on fixed schedules must accommodate the disabled person
B. Canada
  1. There is a duty to accommodate disabled person in most provinces.
  2. Public transportation must accommodate disabled people who work.
■ Vocational rehabilitation assistance
A. Social Security Administration (SSA)
  1. Put individuals in touch with agencies for:
     ✦ job counseling
     ✦ job training
     ✦ job placement
B. Rehabilitation programs services
  1. Ticket to Work and Work Incentive Improvement Act of 1999
C. State Vocational Rehabilitation Agencies
  1. Application
  2. Eligibility
  3. Joint program planning with rehab counselor
  4. Types of vocational rehabilitation services
D. Work incentive programs via SSA, using trial work periods without losing benefits
■ Summary
A. MS care is extremely costly as is the cost of the illness over a lifetime.
B. Adjustments are required to promote continued employment.
C. Disease-modifying therapy, while costly, may result in sustained employment over a lifetime with MS.
D. The goal is to promote independent living with MS with a desired quality of life.

ADDITIONAL READING
Burks JS, Johnson KP, eds., *Multiple Sclerosis: Diagnosis, Treatment, and Rehabilitation*. New York: Demos Medical Publishing, 2001.
Coyle PK, CMSC meeting, Ft. Worth, TX, 2002. Personal communication.
Gulick EE. November 2001. Toronto, Canada. Personal communication.
Northrop D. "Advocacy." In: Halper J, Holland NJ, eds., *Comprehensive Nursing Care in Multiple Sclerosis*, 2nd Ed. New York: Demos Medical Publishing, 2002.

Chapter 18

Primary Care Needs

Objectives:
Upon completion of this chapter, the learner will:

◆ Describe the importance of the maintenance of a balanced health state
◆ Discuss primary care needs in MS
◆ Cite specific wellness activities in MS for men and women

■ Annual physical examinations are essential for men and women with MS.
■ They should include:
  A. Blood work (CBC, comprehensive profile, thyroid function tests)
  B. Height and weight if possible
  C. Blood pressure
  D. Assessment for risk factors (osteoporosis, diabetes, etc.)
  E. Education regarding exercise, smoking, diet, etc.
■ Hormonally mediated events
  A. Pregnancy (there is a 70% reduction in risk of exacerbation during pregnancy and a 70% increase the 3 to 8 months postpartum)
    1. Education should include assessment of:
      ✦ The patient's capabilities before conception
      ✦ Available supports for the postpartum period
      ✦ Considerations regarding breast feeding versus bottle feeding, issues of fatigue, DMAs
      ✦ The family's living situation and economic resources

- Menstrual cycle assessment should include normal cycle, premenstrual syndrome, cramping, bloating, current medications.
- Menopause—there is a paucity of research in this area. Current information about hormone replacement therapy (HRT) is confusing regarding risk reduction for osteoporosis and for coronary heart disease (CHD) and osteoporosis. Consultation with a gynecologist may be recommended.
- Recognizing and preventing pseudoexacerbations should include the following caveats:
  A. Avoid increasing core body temperature (fever).
  B. Maintain body coolness with cooling devices, cool drinks, and cool showers if ambient temperature is high.
  C. Cool down frequently when exercising, and exercise in a cool environment.
  D. Treat infections promptly.
- Osteoporosis
  A. May occur in both men and women with MS
  B. Is associated with reduced mobility and use of corticosteroids
  C. Falls may result in fractures and increased disability
  D. Assessment should include bone density study (DXA); a z-score of less than –2.0 requires treatment
  E. Treatment consists of:
    1. Education about risk reduction and safety measures at home
    2. Exercise is recommended for the prevention and treatment of osteoporosis
    3. Protective pads should be worn around the outer thigh covering the trochanteric region of the hip
    4. Optimal calcium intake with Vitamin D (400 IU for those under 65; 600–800 for those who are older)
    5. Estrogen therapy is controversial at this time (results of the Women's Health Initiative)
    6. SERMs (raloxifene or tamoxifen) may have potential benefit
    7. Bisphosphonates are the drugs of choice
       ✦ aldendronate (daily or weekly)
       ✦ risedronate
       ✦ research studies:
         ✧ calcitonin
         ✧ parathyroid hormone

8. Conclusion—preventing bone loss and vertebral fractures can be attained to some degree with any of the currently approved medications, exercise, and possibly diet. A person who has sustained a fracture is certainly a candidate for pharmacologic therapy.

■ Pulmonary complications

A. Pulmonary dysfunction secondary to MS is a leading cause of morbidity and mortality in MS.

B. Assessment should include history of pneumonia, aspiration, dypnea, weak cough, hypophonia, and fatigue.

C. Treatment is predicated on noninvasive interventions whose goals are to:

1. Prevent respiratory failure
2. Maintain normal lung ventilation
3. Maintain normal lung compliance
4. Help eliminate airway secretions through more-effective cough flow
5. Avoid upper respiratory infections, particularly during the influenza season

ADDITIONAL READING

Halper J. "Women's Issues in Multiple Sclerosis." In: Halper J, ed., *Advanced Concepts in Multiple Sclerosis Nursing Care.* New York: Demos Medical Publishing, 2002; 141–145.

Lehman L, Picone MA. "Pulmonary Complications." In: Halper J, ed., *Advanced Concepts in Multiple Sclerosis Nursing Care.* New York: Demos Medical Publishing, 2002; 137–148.

Nieves JW, Cosman F. Management strategies for osteoporosis. *Emerg Med* July 2002; 37–48.

Chapter 19

The Nurse's Role in MS Research

Objectives:
Upon completion of this chapter, the learner will:

◆ Describe the roles and responsibilities of the nurse in MS research
◆ Identify key concepts in the research process

■ Responsibilities of the research coordinator
 A. Liaison
 B. Facilitator
 C. Educator
 D. Administrator
 E. Recruiter
 F. Advocate
  1. Protecting human rights
  2. Nurturing patient retention
  3. Maintaining regulatory files
  4. Providing accurate documentation
  5. Promoting adherence to the protocol
  6. Clarifying false expectations
  7. Recognizing and reporting adverse events
  8. Inspiring hope
■ Study files notebook includes:
 A. Protocol—all versions
 B. Protocol amendments
 C. Consent forms—all versions
 D. Investigator's brochure
 E. 1572 forms and all updates

    F. Curricula vitae of all those listed in 1572
    G. IRB approvals
    H. IRB membership
    I. IRB correspondence
    J. Safety reports
    K. SAE reports
    L. Laboratory documents (normal values and certificates)
    M. Drug accountability log
    N. Sponsor correspondence
    O. Monitoring log
    P. Enrollment log
- Definition of terms
    A. *Protocol*—a framework for the conduct of the study.
    B. *Investigator's brochure*—a detailed, confidential description of the structure and formulation of the drug, and a summary of the studies and adverse events.
    C. *1572*—the official document that secures the investigator's commitment to conduct the study within FDA guidelines.
    D. *Source documents*—documents that contain all the clinical information gathered during a visit.
    E. *Case report forms*—concise information reflective of the source documents entered into duplicate forms that are collected and returned to the sponsor for data entry.
- Trial design
    A. *Open label*—the investigators and patients are aware of what drug or treatment is being tested.
    B. *Single-blinded study*—the patient is blinded to the treatment but the investigator is aware of what is being tested.
    C. *Double-blinded study*—neither the investigator nor the patient knows who has been randomly assigned to what treatment (active therapy or placebo).
    D. *Cross-over study*—participants receive either placebo or tested therapy over a specific time, then investigational drug for the remainder of the study.
- Institutional Review Board (IRB) determines that:
    A. Risks to subjects are minimized.
    B. Risks to subjects are reasonable in relation to anticipated benefits.
    C. Selection of subjects is equitable.

D. Informed consent is obtained from the subjects or from a legal representative.

E. The research has a rational scientific basis, as does the methodology.

F. The research plan makes adequate provision for monitoring the data to ensure the safety of subjects.

G. There are adequate provisions to protect the privacy of the subject.

■ Informed consent is based on ethical principles of full disclosure and the right of self-determination. The consent must be easily understood by a lay person and must contain the following:

A. A statement that the study involves research

B. An explanation of the purpose of the research, the design or the study, and procedures that are experimental

C. A description of any foreseeable risks or discomforts including, for women who are able to have children, risks to childbearing or to the fetus.

D. A description of potential benefits

E. A disclosure of appropriate alternative procedures or course of treatment, if any, that may be advantageous to the subject

F. A statement describing the extent to which confidentiality of records will be maintained, including the fact that the FDA might inspect the records

G. For research involving more than a minimal risk, an explanation as to whether compensation and medical treatments are available

H. An explanation of who should be contacted for answers to pertinent questions about the research and the research subject's rights

I. A statement that participation is voluntary, refusal to partici-pate will not result in any penalty or loss of service to which the subject is otherwise entitled, and that the subject may withdraw at any time without penalty

■ Adverse events

A. *Adverse drug experience*—any unfavorable and unintended sign, symptom, or disease temporally associated with the use of investigational product

B. *Serious adverse drug experience*—any experience that results in death, a life-threatening adverse event, inpatient hospitalization or prolongation of hospitalization, a persistent or significant disability or incapacity related to the research

C. *Unexpected adverse drug experience*—any adverse experience, the specificity or severity of which is not consistent with the current investigator's brochure

- Nursing assessment
  A. How realistic are the patient's expectations of what the drug under study will and will not do for MS?
  B. Does the person understand that there might be a chance of receiving a placebo (in placebo-controlled studies)?
  C. Is the patient committed to the frequency of visits, testing requirements, and procedures outlined in the consent form and protocol?
  D. How successful has the patient been in the past in terms of keeping appointments and adhering to treatments?
  E. Does the patient lack adequate insurance for currently available treatments?
  F. Is the patient experiencing a decline in functional status despite aggressive therapeutic interventions?

- Recommendations for research nurse coordinators:
  A. A study has a beginning, middle, and end; there will be closure.
  B. Study work will satisfy a compulsive edge, if you have one.
  C. Keep in touch with other nurse coordinators for support and information.
  D. Take care of yourself; this is hard work.
  E. Participate in the investigators' meeting; this is your opportunity to share experiences with others and with the sponsor.
  F. Think of research questions you may want to incorporate into the study; sponsors often are interested in other research questions.

ADDITIONAL READING

Morgante L. "Research Coordinator: Another Dimension of MS Nursing." In: Halper J, ed., *Advanced Concepts in Multiple Sclerosis Nursing Care.* New York: Demos Medical Publishing, 2001; 85–99.

Chapter 20

Study Guide in Multiple Sclerosis

Additional Readings

The Canadian Multiple Sclerosis Nursing Care Plan. Mississauga, Ontario: Intramedical Health Services, 2000.

Bowling AC. *Alternative Medicine and Multiple Sclerosis.* New York: Demos, 2001.

Burks JS, Johnson KP, eds. *Multiple Sclerosis: Diagnosis, Medical Management, and Rehabilitation.* New York: Demos, 2002.

Cassidy CA. Using the transtheoretical model to facilitate behavior change in patients with chronic illness. *J Am Acad Nurse Practit* 1999; 11(7):281–287.

Cook S, ed. *Handbook of Multiple Sclerosis.* 3rd ed. New York: Marcel Decker, 2001.

Coyle PK, Halper J. *Meeting the Challenge of Progressive Multiple Sclerosis.* New York: Demos, 2001.

Goldberg S. *Clinical Neuroanatomy Made Ridiculously Simple.* Miami: Med Master, 1979.

Holland NJ, Murray TJ, Reingold SC. *Multiple Sclerosis: A Guide for the Newly Diagnosed.* New York: Demos, 2001.

Holland NJ, Halper J, eds., *Multiple Sclerosis: A Self-Care Guide to Wellness.* Washington, D.C. Paralyzed Veterans of America, 1998.

Kalb RC, ed. *Multiple Sclerosis: The Questions You Have—The Answers You Need.* New York: Demos, 2000.

Kalb RC, ed., *Multiple Sclerosis: A Guide for Families.* New York: Demos, 1998.

Lublin FD, Reingold SC. Defining the course of multiple sclerosis: Results of an international survey. *Neurology* 1996, 46:907–911.

Multiple Sclerosis Council for Clinical Practice Guidelines. *Urinary Dysfunction and Multiple Sclerosis.* Evidence-based management strategies for urinary dysfunction in multiple sclerosis. Washington, D.C. Paralyzed Veterans Association, 1999.

Paty D, Ebers GC, eds. *Multiple Sclerosis.* Philadelphia: FA Davis, 1998.

Polman, CH, et al. *Multiple Sclerosis: The Guide to Treatment and Management,* 5th ed. New York: Demos, 2001.

Rao SM, Leo GJ, Bernardin L, Unverzagt F. Cognitive dysfunction in multiple sclerosis. I. Frequency, patterns, and prediction. *Neurology* 1991; 41:685–691.

Rudick R, Goodkin D, eds. *Multiple Sclerosis Therapeutics.* London: Martin Dunitz, 1999.

Rumrill PD. *Employment Issues in Multiple Sclerosis.* New York: Demos, 1996.

Schapiro RT. *Symptom Management in Multiple Sclerosis.* New York: Demos, 1998.

Sheehan G, Barnes MP, eds. *Spasticity Rehabilitation.* London: Churchill Communications Europe, 1998.

The Multiple Sclerosis Nurse Specialist Consensus Committee. *Multiple Sclerosis: Key Issues in Nursing Management: Adherence, Cognitive Function, Quality of Life.* Columbia, MD: Medicalliance, 1998.

The Multiple Sclerosis Nurse Specialist Consensus Committee. *Best Practices in Nursing Care: Disease Management, Pharmacological Treatment, Nursing Research.* Columbia, MD: Medicalliance, 2000.

Thompson A, Polman C, Hohlfeld R, eds. *Multiple Sclerosis: Clinical Challenges and Controversies.* London: Martin Dunitz, 1997.

van den Noort S, Holland NJ, eds. *Multiple Sclerosis in Clinical Practice.* New York: Demos, 1999.

Zorzon M, Zivadinov R, Boxco A, et al. Sexual dysfunction in multiple sclerosis: A case-control study. I. Frequency and comparison of groups. *Multiple Sclerosis* 1999; 5(6):418–427.

Chapter 21

Case Studies

Case Study 1

Sally is thirty-four years old and was diagnosed with MS in 1992. She initially experienced a relapsing-remitting course in which her exacerbations were mild and occurred infrequently. After her second pregnancy, about 6 months postpartum, she had a severe exacerbation that resulted in paralysis of both lower extremities. Following hospitalization for intravenous steroids, she was treated in an inpatient rehabilitation hospital for strengthening and improvement of function. When she was discharged, she was able to walk with a wheeled walker and she used a motorized tricart for longer distances.

Her ability to walk has diminished, she is able to stand and pivot for transfers, and only take a few steps to and from chairs and her bed. She continues to experience attacks of her MS and, despite treatment with steroids, she has had incomplete recovery (secondary progressive MS). She requires maximal assistance to get in and out of her car. She uses a tub transfer chair to bathe and grab bars to get up and down from her commode. She uses a long-handled reacher in her kitchen and bedroom to reach items on high shelves. She has had a ramp installed at her front door and has widened the doorways in her home to accommodate her scooter. She is subject to fatigue and finds that if she rests in the afternoons, she is able to stay up until 9 or 10 PM before going to bed.

Sally and her family have had frequent contact with the National Multiple Sclerosis Society (NMSS), participating in several educational programs, family weekends, and support groups. Sally receives her care at an MS Center where, in addition to neurologic care, she has had nursing care for bladder and bowel management, counseling to assist her to adjust to her changing physical condition, and rehabilitation services. She has had physical therapy for mobility and to develop a home program, and occupational therapy for upper extrem-

Answers to the questions asked in these case studies can be found on page 112.

ity function and the appropriate use of assistive devices. Her current medications consist of Ditropan® and Hiprex® for her bladder, Cylert® for fatigue, and Neurontin® for pain. Sally's condition continues to worsen and her neurologist has discussed immunomodulating therapy, but has not suggested a particular product. Sally is unsure about what to do and comes to you for advice and education.

1. What should one consider in assisting Sally with her decision regarding therapy?
    a. Cost of therapy and her insurance coverage
    b. Efficacy of the proposed treatment and tolerability
    c. Her ability to manage the proposed therapy
    d. Impact on her quality of life
    e. All of the above

2. What types of education will Sally and her family need should she decide to begin therapy?
    a. Reconstitution and injection of medication
    b. Managing side effects
    c. What she can expect from therapy
    d. How others have managed
    e. All of the above
    f. a, b, and d

3. What strategies have shown to facilitate adherence to complex protocols (select all that apply)?
    a. Assisting patients with injections until they are able to accomplish the task
    b. A strong health provider/patient relationship
    c. One good educational session
    d. A supportive social network

4. Sally has occasional short-term memory problems, particularly when she is fatigued. How can you overcome this deficit and facilitate adherence?
    a. Give simple, structured instructions
    b. Reinforce the material frequently
    c. Involve care partners in the care
    d. Provide written material
    e. All of the above

Case Study 2

Roberta is a fifty-five-year-old woman with a twenty-two-year history of multiple sclerosis. In the early 1980s she began to experience gradual weakness in her legs, and was using a walker by 1985. She showed signs of spasticity in her legs at that time and was started on a low dose of oral baclofen. Over time, she became weaker and the spasticity worsened. She began using increasing doses of oral baclofen with some symptom relief. By 1994, she was triplegic and experiencing severe neurogenic bowel and bladder dysfunction. By 1997, she was unable to feed herself, her speech was hypophonic, and she needed a highly regimented bladder and bowel management program. She became increasing fatigued, forgetful, and withdrawn. She was taking baclofen 160 mg per day, and Zanaflex® was added starting with 2 mg. hs. Roberta's physician had suggested that she consider an intrathecal pump for delivery of baclofen but she refused.

1. The benefits of intrathecal delivery of baclofen include:
   a. Lower doses
   b. Minimal systemic absorption
   c. Lower cost
   d. Improved cognitive function
   e. All of the above

2. Intrathecal baclofen is only used for nonambulatory patients.
   a. True
   b. False
   c. Not sure

3. Patient and family education should include the following:
   a. Responsibilities of the patient and family
   b. Refills and dosage changes
   c. Potential risks and benefits of intrathecal baclofen
   d. Implications on other symptoms of MS
   e. All of the above

4. The most influential factor in choosing intrathecal baclofen might be:
   a. Postsurgical quality of life
   b. Impact on cognitive status
   c. General health state
   d. Insurance coverage

Case Study 3

William is a thirty-five-year-old executive who works 50 to 60 hours per week and travels frequently. He has a seven-year history of MS. Initially, he had infrequent exacerbations which were treated with short courses of either intravenous or oral steroids. Two years ago he developed bilateral lower extremity weakness, a T10 sensory level, and forgetfulness. Treatment was begun with Copaxone®, which he uses only intermittently because he does not see himself "getting better." He has difficulty with self-injection but is reluctant to ask his family for assistance.

William has become increasingly anxious. His social situation and work have suffered and he is becoming more isolated.

1. The treatment approach for this patient should include:
   a. Discussion of psychosocial concerns
   b. Review of his treatment expectations
   c. Counseling regarding energy conservation and vocational activities
   d. Changing his immunomodulating agent
   e. a, b, and c

2. In addition, other appointments should be scheduled for (check all that apply):
   a. Vocational counseling and retraining
   b. Physical therapy for exercise and gait training
   c. Counseling for loss of physical abilities, altered life style, and occupational difficulties
   d. Discussion of long-term disability benefits
   e. Family meeting
   f. All of the above

Case Study 4

Kenneth is a forty-two-year-old man with a ten-year history of relapsing-remitting MS. He is no longer working due to cognitive changes resulting from MS. He had experienced two relapses during the past year, and both he and his wife are anxious to begin a disease modifying agent as soon as possible. Kenneth is interested in injecting himself, but his wife had concerns about his ability to learn this technique.

1. What educational strategies will assist this couple in learning an injectable procedure?
   a. Audio and video material along with written instructions
   b. Watching another patient self-inject
   c. Demonstrating the technique to the nurse during one office visit
   d. Having a visiting nurse teach the patient and wife at home
   e. a, c, and d

2. Adherence can be promoted by:
   a. Calling the patient regularly after he begins self-injection
   b. Asking that he keep records of his injection sites
   c. Asking his wife to monitor him regularly
   d. Referring him to a network of patients using the same medication
   e. Schedule follow-up appointment in 2 to 3 months after starting injections
   f. All of the above

Case Study 5

Maryann is a twenty-seven-year-old woman with a three-year history of relapsing-remitting multiple sclerosis. She has had four relapses since her diagnosis and has recovered completely from all but the last relapse, which left her with sensory deficits in both feet. She works full-time as a legal secretary and enjoys an active social life. Maryann is concerned about her incomplete recovery after her last relapse and wants to begin one of the new disease-modifying agents. Her neurologist presented her with all available treatment options, but felt that she should select the treatment that would best fit her lifestyle.

1. Education about available treatments should be provided in a therapeutic environment which includes:
   a. Patient and healthcare providers
   b. Other MS patients and their families
   c. One-to-one interactions
   d. All of the above

2. Treatment decisions should be based on:
   a. Tolerability
   b. Impact upon quality of life
   c. Efficacy
   d. All of the above

3. The goal of patient and family education in multiple sclerosis is to:
   a. Promote informed decision making
   b. Cure the patient's problems
   c. Substantiate the need for nursing care
   d. Reduce healthcare costs

Case Study 6

Martin, a twenty-three-year-old with a five-year history of multiple sclerosis, developed vertigo and incoordination of gait over a seven-day period, which stabilized and slowly improved over the next month. Two years later the symptoms returned, along with ill-defined difficulty with blurred vision, which also improved when a course of intravenous steroids was given. Within the next year he began to note severe spasticity of his lower extremities with resultant problems with gait, transfers, and bed mobility. Treatment with baclofen and Zanaflex® resulted in minimal improvement. His motor and cerebellar symptoms progressed and he was nonambulatory at age twenty five. He was seen at the MS Center complaining of pain and rigidity in his legs, bowel and bladder incontinence, and anxiety. He reported no cognitive difficulties. Martin is requesting treatment with immunomodulating therapy.

1. What is the treatment priority for this patient?
   a. Spasticity management
   b. Injectable therapies
   c. Counseling/education
   d. Clarification of treatment goals as related to quality of life

2. Injectable therapy is indicated in light of this patient's condition and history.
   a. True
   b. False
   c. Not sure

3. What additional interventions does this patient require at this time?
   a. Confirm that the patient understands his current health state
   b. Evaluate and enhance his support systems
   c. Start a rehabilitation program
   d. All of the above

Case Study 7

Felicia lives alone. Her daughter is away at college. Her husband left her about one year ago for another woman. She has secondary progressive MS and has minimal household assistance. She is fiercely independent yet is exposed to household dangers (cooking, toileting, bathing). She was hospitalized in August for an acute exacerbation (right arm weakness and increased tremor), then sent to subacute rehabilitation. She made little progress and was advised that it would be safer for her to consider long-term living options (assisted living, nursing home) rather than return home. She refused and returned to her home with 2 hours of home health aide assistance three times a week. She calls the MS Center three or four times a week with questions and concerns (What medications am I on? I dropped my pills— I need more. I have no food in the house.) She still refuses to discuss living elsewhere.

1. What are the primary concerns for this patient?
   a. Safety issues
   b. Socialization concerns
   c. Emotional reaction to MS

2. What would be the most therapeutic intervention for this patient?
   a. Contacting public health department in her town
   b. Counseling the patient about dangers in her home
   c. Continuing to support her in her decision
   d. Telling the patient to seek care elsewhere

3. What are the cognitive issues in this situation?
   a. Impaired judgment
   b. Poor executive function
   c. Rigidity
   d. All of the above

4. What are the emotional reactions that an MS nurse might experience with this patient?
   a. Anger
   b. Frustration
   c. Hopefulness
   d. a and b only
   e. a, b, and c

Case Study 8

Helen is a forty-six-year-old woman with a twenty-five-year history of multiple sclerosis. She is wheelchair-confined and has severe tremor. Her husband is a house painter and is away all day. Helen has two young children (12 and 10) who are doing very poorly in school and who are not supervised in the afternoon. She sleeps a great deal during the day and is up most of the night. Her husband complains that he is unable to sleep and rest because of his wife's sleep patterns. She has emotional outbursts, screaming at her family for minimal infractions of "the rules" and is emotionally labile with unexpected crying jags. The children are having problems in school with homework, interpersonal relations, and cleanliness. The husband is overwhelmed and does not understand the problem. He feels his wife could do better if she tried.

1. What education and information will help this family at this time?
   a. Discussion of cognitive impairments and MS
   b. Description of how MS has affected Helen
   c. Agreeing with husband that the patient can do better if she tried
   d. a and b only

2. What services are important to this family at this time?
   a. A home health aide for Helen
   b. Placement in a long-term facility
   c. Assistance with the children when they return from school
   d. None of the above
   e. a and c

3. What mental/social services health services might be helpful at this time?
   a. Neuropsychological evaluation
   b. Psychiatric evaluation
   c. Home health evaluation
   d. All of the above

4. Emotional lability has been associated with multiple sclerosis.
   a. True
   b. False

Case Study 9

Thomas has been married to Theresa for twenty years. She has had MS for nineteen years and was initially very stable. She worked until two years ago and raised two children, both of whom are now in college. Theresa has become increasingly disabled during the past two years. She uses a walker in the house and a wheelchair outdoors. She is no longer able to do laundry, prepare meals, or manage the house (shopping, cleaning, pay bills) due to fatigue, forgetfulness, and problems with her handwriting. Frequently, when Thomas returns home from work, Theresa is sitting watching TV. She has soiled herself yet is unaware of her incontinence. Thomas is then faced with the tasks of cleaning her (and the furniture), preparing dinner, doing household tasks, and assisting Theresa with her personal hygiene before bed. He complains of having no life and no one to talk to. He complains of disturbance in his sleep patterns (Theresa occasionally wanders at night and has to be assisted to the bathroom), decreased appetite, and a feeling of hopelessness. He is concerned about burdening his children.

1. What nursing intervention would be appropriate at this time?
   a. Advising Thomas to obtain personal assistance for his wife
   b. Encouraging Thomas to place his wife in a long-term facility
   c. Advising Thomas to use diapers for his wife
   d. Informing Thomas that this is all part of MS

2. What assessments might be helpful at this time?
   a. Neuropsychological screening
   b. Comprehensive rehabilitation evaluation at home
   c. Vocational assessment
   d. a and b only

3. What assistance can you offer Thomas to help him cope with his wife's advancing disability?
   a. Counseling by a mental health professional
   b. A men's support group
   c. Education about multiple sclerosis and personalized information about his wife
   d. Encouragement to continue to cope with the current situation

4. What nursing interventions might improve the patient's symptomatic problems?
   a. Bowel management program
   b. Assessment of bladder function
   c. Review of patient's medications
   d. All of the above

Case Study 10

Gerald is a forty-two-year-old man with a ten-year history of multiple sclerosis. He is married, has three children ages 14, 12, and 8. He served in the Navy prior to his marriage and then became a security guard at a local company. He has brainstem symptoms (tremor, ataxia, nystagmus) and is no longer able to work. He has a gun collection in his home. He has been hospitalized three times during the past five years for paranoid behaviors. Following his most recent hospitalization, he promised that he would remove the guns from his home. He has been tested for cognitive impairment (memory, judgment, and learning have been affected) and has been counseled by a neuropsychologist until his insurance ceased covering for care.

He has become increasingly abusive to his wife and family as his condition has progressed. He threatens his wife and children with both physical abuse and with his guns. He is intermittently depressed and exhibits paranoid behaviors (his wife is having an affair, his daughter should have been an abortion). He uses foul language in front of his children. Recently, his wife has been participating in counseling; the patient refuses to do so. She has returned to work since finances are a problem in light of the needs of the growing children. Gerald has told his home health aide that he plans to kill his wife. The children are having problems in school; they are responsible for the patient's care when they return home in the afternoons.

1. What is the first step for the nurse upon hearing this information?
   a. Discuss the situation with patient's wife
   b. Try to reason with the patient
   c Inform nursing supervisor
   d. Inform the patient's physician immediately
   e. Contact the authorities
   f. All of the above

g. a, c, d, and e

h. a, c, d

i. None of the above

2. Should the patient agree to hospitalization, what discharge planning would be helpful for this family?
   a. Ongoing assessment and treatment by a mental health professional
   b. Support groups for his wife and children
   c. Day treatment program for the patient
   d. All of the above

3. Would neuropsychological reassessment be helpful at this time?
   a. Yes
   b. No

4. What other nursing interventions would be helpful upon the patient's discharge?
   a. Patient and family education about the emotional aspects of MS
   b. Advising the family to consider long-term placement if this situation continues to worsen
   c. Ensuring that the home environment is safe for the patient and family
   d. All of the above

Answers to Case Study Questions

Case Study 1
1. e
2. e
3. b
4. e

Case Study 2
1. e
2. b
3. e
4. a

Case Study 3
1. e
2. f

Case Study 4
1. e
2. f

Case Study 5
1. d
2. d
3. a

Case Study 6
1. c
2. b
3. d

Case Study 7
1. a
2. c
3. d
4. b

Case Study 8
1. d
2. e
3. d
4. a

Case Study 9
1. a
2. d
3. c
4. d

Case Study 10
1. g
2. d
3. a
4. d

Chapter 22

Certification Study Questions

1. Which of the following statements about the possible cause(s) of MS is incorrect?
   a. Abnormal autoimmune response to myelin develops after exposure to some environmental agent in genetically predisposed individuals
   b. Immune system activation
   c. Decreased production of inflammatory cytokines
   d. Combined effects of the autoimmune response cause the demyelination, axonal damage, and scarring seen in patients with MS

2. Onset of MS usually occurs in persons who are ages:
   a. 20–40
   b. 40–50
   c. 10–30
   d. 30–50

3. How many exacerbations, with neurologic symptoms referable to lesions in the white matter of the CNS, must a patient experience before a definite diagnosis of MS can be made?
   a. One
   b. Two
   c. Three
   d. Four

4. On onset, MS follows a relapsing-remitting pattern in approximately what percentage of patients?
   a. 50
   b. 85
   c. 30
   d. 15

5. Continuing care needs of a patient with relapsing-remitting MS do not include:
   a. Ensuring adequate access to medications and adaptive equipment

   b. Encouraging sustained treatment with a disease-modifying agent

   c. Discouraging patient autonomy

   d. Monitoring patient's self-care abilities

6. Sustaining care for patients with advanced MS may include all *except* which of the following?

   a. Interventions to prevent pressure sores

   b. Providing palliative care

   c. Recommending installation of adaptive hand controls on the patient's automobile

   d. Providing information and counseling regarding advance directives

7. Which of the following agents reduce relapse rates in MS?

   a. Benzodiazepines

   b. Glatiramer acetate

   c. IV methylprednisolone

   d. All of the above

8. Agents that may help reduce symptoms of fatigue include all of the following *except*:

   a. Pemoline

   b. Methyphidate

   c. Clonazepam

   d. Modafinil

9. Interferons and glatiramer acetate should be started early in the disease because they do all of the following *except*:

   a. Slow progression of the disease

   b. Reduce relapses

   c. Cure MS

   d. May delay progression of disability

10. Which of the following complications should a nurse caring for a patient with advanced MS be alert to?

   a. Pressure ulcers

   b. Difficulty swallowing

   c. Depression

   d. All of the above

11. As part of continuing care for patients with relapsing-remitting MS who have experienced a relapse, the nurse will need to do all of the following *except*:

   a. Emphasize the importance of continuing treatment

b. Reassess the treatment regimen

c. Advise the patient to take a drug holiday

d. Help the patient to establish realistic expectations of the drug therapy

12. Which of the following statements about the role of MS nurses is not correct?

    a. Cost containment pressures brought about a dramatic and ongoing expansion in the role of the nurse

    b. Nurses have had decreasing prescriptive authority

    c. The MS nurse provides primary, acute, specialized, and rehabilitative care for patients with multiple sclerosis

    d. Nurses provide education, support, and healthcare delivery for patients and their families

13. All of the following characterize the aims of nursing research *except*:

    a. Generate new knowledge

    b. Validate existing knowledge

    c. Guide nursing practice

    d. Diagnose MS

14. Nurses who wish to conduct research can begin to seek funding and support by:

    a. Identifying funding sources

    b. Developing grant-writing skills

    c. Identifying and developing collaborative relationships

    d. All of the above

15. Which of the following statements about MS is correct?

    a. Life expectancy from time of diagnosis is generally 10 years

    b. The age of onset is 40–60 years

    c. MS affects more women than men

    d. The recent development of a cure for MS has brought hope to patients and their families

16. Which of the following statements about the pathophysiology of MS is true?

    a. The lesions associated with MS are particularly prevalent in the optic nerves and the gray matter of the spinal cord, brainstem, cerebellum, and cerebrum

    b. Loss of the myelin sheath disrupts electrical conduction within the CNS

    c. MS is thought to occur secondary to a bacterial infection

    d. Myelin loss occurs only in the spinal cords of people with MS

17. Which of the following statements about MS is not true?
   a. People with MS frequently experience neurologic deficits such as tremor, sensory loss, and bladder incontinence
   b. Secondary symptoms of MS include bladder infections and pressure sores
   c. Cognitive impairment in people with MS occurs only rarely
   d. Neurologic signs and symptoms associated with MS are dependent on the location of the lesions in the CNS

18. Which of the following statements about MS is correct?
   a. MRI is the gold standard used to definitely diagnose MS
   b. Evoked potential testing is not helpful in the diagnosis of MS
   c. In approximately 85% of people with MS, the course is described as relapsing-remitting at the time of diagnosis
   d. The course of MS is invariably characterized by progressive deterioration

19. Which of the following statements is not true?
   a. Four disease-modifying agents have been approved in relapsing-remitting MS
   b. IFNB-1b is an immunomodulating agent
   c. Glatiramer acetate's mode of action involves inhibition of the immune response to myelin basic protein and other myelin antigens
   d. IFNB-1a is only administered intramuscularly

20. Which of the following statements is correct?
   a. Adherence to medications is independent of sex, age, and other demographics
   b. Information should imply that there is no real risk associated with MS with or without treatment
   c. Healthcare professionals should always be in charge of making decisions about treatment
   d. People who think that their disease is not under their control adhere more readily to treatment

21. You are caring for a patient with relapsing-remitting MS who has just started treatment with interferon therapy. Which information is least likely to facilitate adherence?
   a. Interferon reduces the frequency of exacerbations but does not restore function
   b. Interferon can be associated with unpleasant side effects
   c. Interferon can be associated with unpleasant side effects but these must be weighed against potential benefits

  d. Patients are encouraged to self-administer interferons

22. Which of the following is not generally considered a barrier to adherence?
  a. Lack of knowledge
  b. Overly optimistic expectations
  c. Lack of financial support
  d. Age

23. Which of the following statements is not correct?
  a. Patient satisfaction has no effect on adherence
  b. Empathizing with patients facilitates adherence
  c. Cultural differences can influence adherence
  d. Problems with reasoning can interfere with adherence

24. Which of the following statements is incorrect?
  a. The severity of cognitive impairment varies from patient to patient
  b. Many people with MS retire from work early because of physical and/or cognitive impairments
  c. Cognitive impairment affects more than 75% of persons with MS
  d. Relatively mild and subtle cognitive deficits may have an impact on patients' lives

25. Which of the following cognitive functions is least likely to be affected in people with MS?
  a. Recall memory
  b. Recognition memory
  c. Information processing
  d. Attention and concentration

26. Which of the following statements is correct?
  a. The prevalence of MS-related cognitive impairment is estimated to be less than 20%
  b. Studies using sensitive neuropsychologic instruments suggest that approximately half of the MS population experience cognitive dysfunction
  c. Until recently, the prevalence of cognitive impairment in people with MS was overestimated
  d. Studies using sensitive neuropsychologic instruments suggest that approximately 80% of the MS population experience cognitive dysfunction

27. Which of the following statements is correct?
  a. People with minimal sensory and motor impairment are not at risk of cognitive impairment

   b. A high correlation between the extent of cognitive impair-
      ment and indices of disability has not been demonstrated
   c. Cognitive and neurologic deficits develop in parallel
   d. There is a strong positive correlation between disease course
      and the development of cognitive impairment

28. In which of the following scenarios is neuropsychologic evalua-
    tion not indicated?
    a. An employer reports that a patient is not working as produc-
       tively as he had been
    b. A baseline assessment of cognitive function is desired prior to
       initiating immunomodulating therapy
    c. A family is concerned that a patient may have cognitive
       impairment, but the patient denies any problems and there is
       no clinical evidence for such impairment
    d. The patient reports cognitive deficits that, although subtle or
       fluctuating, may have functional impact

29. Which of the following strategies is unlikely to help patients
    with severe cognitive deficits?
    a. Insight-oriented psychotherapy
    b. Family counseling
    c. Audiotaping information
    d. Minimizing distractions

30. Which of the following is probably the best approach that nurs-
    es can adopt when addressing quality of life issues with people
    with MS?
    a. Nurses should encourage patients to aim for a higher quality
       of life
    b. Nurses should recognize that each patient may have different
       expectations and aspirations
    c. Nurses should constantly re-evaluate the patient's quality of life
    d. It is important to use quality of life questionnaires before ini-
       tiating conversations about quality of life

31. Which of the following statements is correct?
    a. The degree of disability is the sole determinant of quality of
       life in MS
    b. Recognizing the need to respond to change is more important
       than the ability to socialize in MS
    c. Impaired cognition does not affect quality of life
    d. Developing and sustaining satisfying relationships is an
       important factor in MS

32. In general terms, which of the following would be least likely to influence a person's quality of life in MS?
    a. Cognitive deficits
    b. Difficulty walking
    c. Swallowing problems
    d. Family strain

33. The symptoms of multiple sclerosis result from:
    a. Inadequate lymphocyte production
    b. Proliferation of myelin
    c. Inadequate inflammatory response
    d. Demyelination and scarring of nerve fibers

34. Which of the following statements describes the process termed "molecular mimicry?"
    a. The immune system fails to react to a foreign substance
    b. Lymphocytes release antibodies in response to an antigen
    c. The foreign target and the self-target of the immune system share molecular features
    d. An inflammatory process up-regulates adhesion molecules on endothelial cells

35. A patient asks about the purpose of a lumbar puncture. Which of these responses do you make?
    a. Analysis of cerebrospinal fluid is helpful when the results of other tests are inconclusive
    b. If your cerebrospinal fluid is negative, it will confirm that you do not have MS
    c. Examining your cerebrospinal fluid will help us predict the course of your disease
    d. A positive result from the cerebrospinal fluid is a definitive test for MS

36. Which of the following patients has the most favorable prognosis?
    a. 32-year-old woman with ataxia and dysarthria
    b. 28-year-old man with nystagmus and tremor
    c. 42-year-old man with frequent polyregional attacks
    d. 40-year-old woman with MS since 28, with monoregional attacks with two pregnancies

37. All of the following suggest MS *except*:
    a. Gait disturbance
    b. Optic neuritis
    c. Negative Babinski reflex
    d. Presence of Lhermitte's sign

38. In a patient with MS you observe tremors, nystagmus, and ataxia. These symptoms are related to the:
    a. Optic nerve
    b. Brainstem
    c. Spinal cord
    d. Sensory pathways

39. In contrast to interferon therapy, glatiramer acetate:
    a. Has a higher incidence of laboratory abnormalities
    b. Is effective for secondary progressive MS
    c. Is not associated with flu-like symptoms
    d. Can result in long-term side-effects

40. In patients who are being treated with steroids, side effects to report include:
    a. Thirst
    b. Heartburn
    c. Dyspnea
    d. Palpitations
    e. All of the above

41. When assessing a patient who complains of cognitive difficulties, which of the following would you expect to see?
    a. Impaired long-term memory
    b. Decreased general intelligence
    c. Impaired language
    d. Decreased short-term memory

42. In a woman age 32 who has had MS for 3 years, the risks of pregnancy can be explained as follows:
    a. Pregnancy will accelerate the course of your disease
    b. You may experience an exacerbation during pregnancy
    c. Pregnancy has no long-term effect on your disease course but you may have an exacerbation in the postpartum months
    d. Your disease may become secondary progressive during pregnancy

43. Why should people with MS be screened for depression?
    a. People with MS have a higher rate of suicide
    b. Signs of depression can indicate an acceleration of the disease process
    c. Depression can interfere with the effectiveness of medications
    d. Depression is an unusual and serious sign in MS

44. When assessing a patient with MS, which of the following is a primary symptom:
    a. Visual changes
    b. Urinary tract infection
    c. Skin breakdown
    d. Social isolation

45. Which intervention would be most effective to decrease the intensity of MS symptoms?
    a. Warm baths
    b. Aerobic exercise
    c. Well-balanced nutrition
    d. Use of an air conditioner

46. Spasticity management should include the following outcome:
    a. Increased coordination
    b. Decreased fatigue
    c. Increased strength
    d. Decreased clonus

47. Which of the following would indicate that the patient has bladder dysfunction?
    a. I void every four hours
    b. I have difficulty getting up from a chair
    c. I sleep through the night
    d. I have to use a pad to catch my urine

48. Which of these instructions would you give to a patient who is experiencing bowel dysfunction?
    a. The anticholinergic medication that you are taking will decrease constipation
    b. Exercising your anal sphincter will give you bowel control
    c. You should increase your intake of fluids and fiber
    d. Diarrhea is common in MS

49. In a patient experiencing fatigue, instructions should include:
    a. Increased fluids
    b. Avoidance of alcohol
    c. Regular rest periods
    d. Avoidance of exercise

50. When teaching a patient who has cognitive impairment due to MS, all of the following are appropriate *except*:
    a. Playing background music
    b. Using repetition
    c. Encouraging use of lists
    d. Teaching in a familiar setting

Answers to Certification Questions

1. c	26.b
2. a	27. b
3. b	28. b
4. b	29. a
5. c	30. b
6. c	31. d
7. a	32. c
8. c	33. d
9. c	34. c
10. d	35. a
11. c	36. d
12. b	37. c
13. d	38. b
14. d	39. c
15. c	40. e
16. b	41. c
17. c	42. c
18. c	43. a
19. d	44. a
20. a	45. d
21. b	46. d
22. d	47. d
23. a	48. c
24. c	49. c
25. a	50. a